Living Systema – Matt Hill

A guide to getting out of the chair, out of the gym and back to a natural level of health, skill, fitness and wellbeing.

Mirador Publishing
10 Greenbrook Terrace
Taunton
Somerset
TA1 1UT

WARNING

The exercises, ideas, and suggestions in this book are not intended as a substitute for professional medical advice. Always consult your physician or health care professional before beginning any new exercise technique or exercise program, particularly if you are pregnant or nursing, if you are elderly, or if you have any chronic or recurring medical or psychological conditions. Any application of the exercises, ideas, and suggestions in this book is at the reader's sole discretion and risk.

The author and publisher of this book and their employers and employees make no warranty of any kind in regard to the content of this book including, but not limited to, any implied warranties of merchantability, or fitness for any particular purpose. The author and publisher of this book and their employers and employees are not liable or responsible to any person or entity for any errors contained in this document, or for any special, incidental, or consequential damage caused or alleged to be caused directly or indirectly by the information contained in this book.

CONTENTS

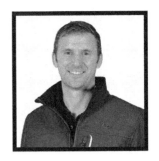

About the Author.

Matt Hill is the owner of his Systema Academy in Wiltshire in the UK. He started training in the Martial Arts in 1987 and by 1991 was living as a full time student of the famous Aikido Teacher Morihiro Saito Sensei in Iwama, Japan, where he lived for two years.

Matt began his study of Systema in 2003. Matt is a qualified Systema Instructor under Vladimir Vasiliev, a 5th Degree black belt in Aikido and an ex Parachute Regiment Captain.

He teaches full time at his Systema Academy as well as leading seminars throughout the UK, and around the world. He is the author of two other books: Systema Health and Systema Combat and a video channel on Pivotshare. He is committed to his personal training and sharing the gift of Systema with as many people as possible.

For more information, complimentary newsletters, details on seminars, training camps and instructional materials please visit:
www.matthill.co.uk

Acknowledgements.

It is difficult to adequately put into words my thanks to Mikhail Ryabko and Vladimir Vasiliev for their guidance. On a daily basis they continue to develop themselves and the System that they have created. Their passion to share this art continues to inspire me and the deeper I study the more I see their genius. The generosity with which they share their art is humbling.

I further extend that thanks to the global Systema community. It grows day by day and wherever I go, the people that I meet are open and friendly.

I also wish to thank my students at the Systema Academy who turn up night after night to train. They mean more to me than they could know and I thank them from the bottom of my heart for allowing me to share with them my love and passion for Systema.

Lastly I would like to thank my wife Sarah, for her help with the manuscript and making it readable. Without her, it would still be sitting in that, 'To Do' list on top of the other two books!

Introduction.

We live in an increasingly fast paced and time-pressured world. Time is the one of those things that we all have in the same amount. Everyone has 24 hours in his or her day. How we spend that time is up to us. How **you** spend your time is of course up to you. This book is not a time management book as such. Instead, it deals with finding everyday moments and actions to train and improve your health, wellbeing and skill.

Some readers may be wondering what Systema is. It simply means: 'The System' in Russian. Systema is a Russian Martial Art. But that description does not come close to explaining what it really is. It needs something else to fully grasp its ability to transform the lives, health and wellbeing of its practitioners. I am not going to go into a long explanation as to what Systema is and its history. Firstly, because that is so hard, and secondly because it doesn't actually matter. It is not a requirement that you understand Systema's history for you to read and benefit from this book.

Systema has four guiding principles: Breathing, Movement, Relaxation and Posture or Structure. It sounds simple, until you try to embody these moment to moment.

Everyone in Systema gets this concept. In fact, I am sure that all readers gets this. How could you not? Who could deny that these four principles are vital to good health and performance in pretty much any subject? There is however, one word that you can place in front of each of these principles that suddenly makes everything much clearer. 'Conscious'. Everyone breathes and moves of course. Equally everyone relaxes to a certain extent and many talk about the importance of posture. But how many do it consciously, moment to moment? In my experience, very few. These four principles have a huge impact on our health and performance. A large part of this book will concern itself with addressing how to make these four principles more conscious in everyday living.

This book is about the moments and making them count. The more you become aware of the moments, the more you make them count. Because if you miss the moments, you miss your life.

How many of you have heard of the competency cycle? It can be applied to almost any skill. Take driving for example.

- **Unconscious Incompetence**. This is when we are not even aware that we can't perform a task well. If we haven't tried to drive manually we are not even aware that we can't perform a gear change.
- **Conscious Incompetence**: This is the stage when we become aware that we can't do it. When we try to change a gear and realise that we can't.
- **Conscious Competence**: We go though the training and skill acquisition to be able to consciously perform the task. Over time we become smooth gear changers and drivers.
- **Unconscious Competence**: We become so practiced that we can perform the skill without really thinking about it. How often have you got in a car and not been able to recall much of the journey? You did everything unconsciously.

Real improvement in Systema comes when you make these normally unconsciously incompetent principles of breathing, movement, relaxation and posture first conscious, then consciously competent and finally unconsciously habitual. When you bring them to every moment and movement. You need to become conscious of your breathing, especially how often you unconsciously hold your breath. You need to become conscious of how you move, how you walk, run, get up, get down etc. The problem is that we have become numbed by too much comfort. It is too easy not to walk, too easy to sit for so long. It is too easy to be entertained without getting off your backside. Too easy to turn a light on, too easy to turn the heating up. We have become deaf to what our bodies need.

You need to notice how tense/relaxed your muscles are at all times, both during movement and when you are still. Finally you need to notice your posture in every position: lying, standing, walking, running, sitting, kneeling etc. When you can do this, you will start to train in every moment. You won't just be training a few hours a week at class, you will start to *Live Systema*.

This book details 20 ways to bring an awareness of Systema's four principles into everyday activities.

I have created a video for each of the 20 practises that is free for owners of the book. You can view the videos by using this link:
http://www.matthill.co.uk/living-systema

Important note:
It should be noted that they are just illustrative examples. The more creative you can be in terms of adapting them to you and making them yours, the better. They are however, a useful guide that will fit in with the lives of nearly everyone. You will notice that none of the pictures are in a gym location or in gym clothes. They are taken in everyday clothes and in everyday locations and situations.

If you can fill the Unforgiving Minute, with sixty seconds worth of distance run...

I am aware that some of these practises may seem trivial on first read, and you may wonder how you can get any benefit. My answer is that it is not the hours but the minutes that really count. It is not what you do a couple of hours a week at training, but rather what you do in every moment. When you can make every second count as Rudyard Kipling said, then you can really start to make some life changing improvements. For the serious martial artist or sports person, the practises in this book do not replace regular practise of your sport or arts specific skills, but rather complements and enhances them.

There is also a final section on developing your awareness, your survival instinct. I believe that this is ultimately the best self-defence skill that we have.

The difference between 'Living' and 'Exercising'.

Think of a Tiger, do you ever see a tiger doing push ups? Their every movement is training. They live their physicality. The catch is that you have to be a tiger in every moment. How do you achieve that? This book is my answer.

This book is about how to be a tiger in every moment, in a sustainable way, for the rest of your life.

Exercise and fitness habits have changed beyond all recognition in the past 50 years.

Even the word exercise is pretty new. Pre the 1950's very few people 'exercised'.

Exercise has gone from being an ordinary activity that was included in day to day living, to a multi-billion dollar industry, plying us with the latest fads to get fit and healthy. This trend has done anything but get us fit and healthy. Obesity rates are soaring as is heart disease and vascular dementia. As a society, we are a bristling knot of stresses, worries, anxieties and disorders. The type of exercise that people are doing now is having little or no difference on our health. Stress is sky high in gyms. The pressure to look good in front of all the mirrors; to look as good as the person running next to you. The anxiety and guilt if you miss a session, the pressure to go harder, heavier, longer... and for what? The race is long and in Baz Lurhman's words, '...it's only with yourself.' The stress that gyms put on us goes against everything that they are trying to achieve in getting us healthy.

This may be a difficult concept to grasp initially. What is wrong with exercise and gyms you may well ask? There was a time, not that long ago, when 'exercising' didn't even cross our minds. Burning calories, and pumping iron were not part of the vernacular. People walked more, sat less and carried more. In short, people moved much, **much** more. You would hardly ever have seen joggers out running; in fact, people would probably have looked at them a little strangely. There were very few if any gyms apart from in schools, the military, police and sports locations. Even then the gyms looked very different to how they look now. No machines to sit on that neglect your core stabilizing muscles. Just ropes, bars, boxes, benches, balls and mats. People trained movements not muscles.

This book is a call to return to natural healthy living, and through that to restore a natural, healthy, fitness.

We will explore ways to bring this approach into your everyday life. *To make existence our exercise.* To bring exercise into every moment, breath and movement; to enable us to be always working out.

To get an idea of how we will approach this, let's rewind the clock a little:

Born to Move

Most of our time on earth has been spent as hunter-gatherers. Think of the everyday lifestyle of one of our ancestors. We would start the day by waking and getting up off the floor. Yes *up off the floor*. Already a big difference to getting out of bed in terms of the range of the movement. We may then have spent 30 minutes foraging for some wood, squatting, bending (properly), stooping, dragging, breaking and carrying armfuls of wood back to the fire. Then we would then probably have adopted a deep natural squat in making the fire. This all-important squat position, as seen in the picture below, (I will come to this later in the book) would continue during the making of breakfast. Other members of the group may well be foraging for berries or mushrooms, or be off on a hunting party ranging for hours or even days for food. Others may be fetching or carrying water.

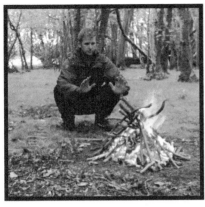

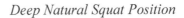
Deep Natural Squat Position

Every year I do one or more outdoor Systema Camps. People don't bring in chairs. Their time is spent standing, walking, working, training, squatting or sitting on the floor or sleeping. It is often a marvel to them to realise that that they have not sat in a chair for a week!

The point is that our daily lives used to contain a huge amount of everyday movement. Nothing too intense or manic, such as a step class, 60 minute run, crossfit or circuit session. This exercise and much more was contained in almost every moment of our existence. It was part of living, not just an hour 2-5 times per week in a gym with fluorescent lighting. There was infinite variety in our movement. We lived in different terrains, weathers, carried varying loads regularly and had to work at varying intensities.

As you will begin to discover in the pages of this book, repeated patterns of movement cause us problems. We wear parts out and we neglect others. *Living exercise* on the other hand, in the real world not in a gym, allows us to be healthy, natural and free, giving us a sustainable healthy life, well into old age. Yes you read that correctly, ***well into old age***.

The current paradigm is that people age badly. There is a decline in people's mobility both in terms of range and amount. Look at the rise of mobility scooters. Vascular dementia is on the rise. When we look at many older people we see the hunched body position of age, where people literally take the position of a chair as seen in the picture below:

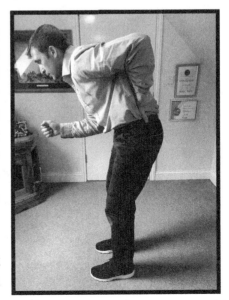

People become very fearful of falling (falling is the biggest cause of death in old age). This fear starts to make them stiff and brittle resulting in even less mobility. It doesn't need to be this way. In previous times people in old age would be taking an active part in everyday life, getting up and down off the floor with ease, walking long distances, doing their share of the work and partaking fully in society. They would be actively engaged right up until the end, when there would be a short period, probably days or weeks of ill health and decreasing mobility before passing. That short period of ill health and decreasing mobility now lasts years or decades in many cases. It doesn't need to be that way.

Health and fitness is not, in my opinion, to be found in a modern gym, under florescent lighting doing repetitive routines a few hours a week. It is to be found in every moment of the day. It is about listening to your body and system and moving much better, and much more. This was how we did it for thousands of years in our past. We were present in our bodies in every moment. This, I believe, is the future of health and fitness.

We need to regain our responsibility for our health and fitness. We need to become more aware of our body, natural awareness, curiosity, spontaneity and sustainability. We can do this by making small changes to the way that we do everyday things. Things that will not be a huge effort, but that gradually pull us back to physicality that should be our birthright. Then, when we obtain it, we will have a lifestyle that will sustain this right to the end.

Systema is a martial art, but not in the sense that many people understand them today. Systema comes from the ages when warriors lived martial arts. A good warrior was a healthy warrior, in mind, body and spirit. This book isn't about teaching you martial arts techniques. It is about changing your attitude and mindset to learning martial arts. To make you healthier, calmer and more aware, in every moment. After all, how often do most of us spend fighting, and I mean real fighting, for our lives? Not very often, if ever hopefully. But all of us live. In every moment. This book is about using those moments to become better at living.

So what should training look like? A good place to start is to ask yourself the question, "What are you trying to get fit for?"

What are you training/getting fit for?

This is a good question. What are your goals? Do you have any?

Most people that have goals are interested in fitness programmes that will have you looking at how far, how fast, how many calories, how much weight, how many reps etc. Note that I am not talking about professional sports people here. Those who are focused or targeted on an event. That training will of course come with specific goals and targets based on their event, although that too has its dangers. At some point they will stop the intensity of their training. When they do, the danger is that many regress into poor levels of health and fitness. You also have to look at how often professionals are injured.

I am talking about everyday people, joining gyms and looking to get fit and healthy generally. Their goals are likely to be based upon training in a gym and in a nutshell improving how they look. But I propose that these are not the best measurements for fitness and health.

What does it matter how many times you can push a bar up and down again?
What does it matter whether you can run 10 miles in under an hour?
What does it matter that you can run 26 miles? The first guy that did this in 490 B.C, Pheidippides of Greece, keeled over and died straight after he passed on his message after the battle of Marathon in Greece!

I would ask the question how do these goals help you in everyday life? This is what I mean when I say what are you fit for.

I understand that personal goals really help people to focus on something and to motivate them to train. But why not make these aspirations more useful? More relevant to the day-to-day aspects of living. How about something like this:

- A pain free body? Not waking up in pain, or feeling your back every time that you bend down, or when getting out of your car after a long journey.
- A body that doesn't get injured so much, that is more resilient to the rigours and demands of everyday life.
- A calm and relaxed mind and body, that is not continuously anxious?
- Having the energy and ability to roll around and play with your children, grandchildren or pets.
- Not groaning when you get out of a chair, up off the floor, or straightening up after digging a patch of soil?
- The freedom and confidence to run down a hill, jump up onto a log and down again, to roll down a slope, climb a tree.
- To be able to fall over, roll and get back up without fear of injury, at any age.

For me, these are natural, human indicators of fitness that should be accessible to **EVERYONE**. Even more than that though, you should move for the pleasure of moving. How it makes you feel. Movement should make you smile. In your whole body. Your body should thank you for it.

In short, how about returning to the physicality you had as a toddler: exquisite mobility and supplety, boundless energy and enthusiasm for movement and play. Just because movement puts a smile on your face. Not stressed because you still have to get so many miles, reps or sessions in this week.

Just because it's mainstream, doesn't mean it's right. Maybe what we need is not to aspire to magazine image fitness or Olympic level performance. Maybe we just need to shed the layers of tension, stiffness, fears and anxieties that life and the years have put on us. To find a joy in just moving freely, much, much more.

My experience is that when you shed the brittleness and tension in the body and find more freedom in movement, you find more freedom of spirit too. As you become more physically confident, you become more emotionally confident. As you become more physically robust, you become more emotionally robust. The two are linked, in our very nature.

For me, it's not rocket science. You just have to move more as our nature intended. Think of the movement involved in socialising and eating around a campfire. You would have to deep squat for long periods, lengthening the lower back, massaging the viscera, strengthening and relaxing the leg muscles.

Sleeping on the floor of a cave or shelter. The simple act of smoothly getting to the ground and up again. Spending a night on the floor comfortably and thus resetting, realigning, and relaxing the joints, muscles and tissues.

Walking long distances everyday to collect water, find wood for the fire and foraging for berries, eggs and other food sources. This would have involved crawling, digging, climbing, dragging, pulling your bodyweight up and over things, lowering your body weight carefully and slowly and carrying varying loads without bags or trolleys.

It is an embarrassment that these should even be things that we are talking seriously about needing to do. It would have been natural for our ancestors. A given. For them purely to exist they would have to do these simplest of human activities. They would not have been part of a fitness program; they were the natural result of the act of being alive and engaged in the world.

The problems with modern day exercise.
There are some real problems with modern day exercise:

- It is too short. We are made to move all day, everyday. We cannot think that a one or two hour window, a couple of times a week, will be enough to compensate for a sedentary lifestyle.
- It is too intense. Exercising like a maniac during these 'short' windows will not make it any better. This adds stress to your system (one of the things that exercising should decrease not increase.) It also dramatically increases the chances of injury.
- The movement range is too limited. Think of the movement patterns involved in the activities in most gyms. Running machines, rowers,

cross-trainers, spin, sitting on weight machines. These are ok as part of a diverse and rounded movement day, but not enough on their own.

- Repetitive movement patterns under fluorescent lighting in air-conditioned rooms. We need and crave variety in our movement. Repetition is at best boring and at worst damaging in that it wears certain parts of the body (think runners knee) and neglects so many other parts of the body.

- It has very little application outside of a gymnasium. Contrived movement patterns will not equate to the random nature of natural movement. If you are training to improve the quality of your life, then you need to move more towards natural movement.

- It has little or no bearing on improving your health or longevity. In fact in the key areas that matter (cardiovascular disease, osteoporosis, cancer, surgeries and life expectancy) there is no difference between exercisers and couch potatoes. Why is this? One reason is because so much of the body's essential movement patterns are neglected.

The coming chapters will explore methods to bring more movement into everyday life. They will help you to bring a moment-to-moment awareness of the state of your health. Your breathing, levels of tension versus relaxation and posture will become moment-to-moment adaptations. They won't require a gym or any equipment, just you and the things around you. Everyday movement is designed to prevent injury and illness, keep us healthy and cure us. My call to action is this: Find more movement in everyday life. Exercise less, move more, move better.

I am passionate that we should not have to suffer unnecessarily in this life. In most cases, people just have to move a little more and a little better.

Before I get onto that however, there is one thing that we have touched on that warrants a little further exploration. ***Overtraining***.

The Dangers of overtraining.

How you feel at the end of a session is the litmus test. You should feel vital and alive, not half dead. You should feel more connected in mind, body and spirit, more resilient and healthier.

If you feel shattered, on your last legs with niggling injuries, most of the time, maybe you need to rethink your training. You are probably also storing up ill health, injury and immobility in old age.

Don't kill yourself every time. We were not designed for it. By all means now and again is good, but all of our systems (immune, digestive, muscular skeletal and nervous to name but four) need balance and rest.

The way that we move is the biggest indicator that we have on the quality of our life. In fact you can say that movement defines our life. The way that someone moves tells us a lot. When they move with ease, smoothness and vitality it tells us a lot about them and the state of their confidence, internal and external health. Equally when someone moves with fear, timidity, injury, effort, lethargy and tension, it also tells us a story.

Nowadays I talk much more about movement sessions than exercise sessions. Easy, relaxed movement is our birthright. We were born to do it and should never not be able to do it. From simple everyday movements such as getting to the floor and back up, ducking under or climbing over something at waist height, crawling under the bed and reversing out or even climbing the stairs. These things should all be done with ease, whatever age you are lucky enough to get to. Equally, climbing a tree, pushing a car, running flat out for

30 seconds or lifting and carrying a heavy object should not be beyond us.

When I teach a Systema class we focus on natural human movement that uses nothing but your body weight, the floor and gravity. Moving your body in every way that it was designed to: running, walking, forwards and backwards, jumping, crawling, throwing, rolling and climbing. Every muscle is used, connected, relaxed and strengthened. When coupled with focus on breathing correctly it is a game changer for your physical and mental wellbeing.

When we move as we were designed, we improve our coordination, digestion, and resilience to injury, boost our immune system and feel happier. We flood our system with a feel good combination of dopamine and serotonin, rather than a stress cocktail of cortisol and adrenaline.

Movement, like life, should be healing, energising, explorative and relaxing to your system. It should be fun, otherwise why do it? Certainly not to lose weight. We all know that losing weight is mostly down to diet don't we? A healthy person should be lean, with loose, long, relaxed muscles easily able to carry their body weight through its complete range of motion.

Movement sessions should also change, regularly bringing in new movements, even small changes to keep the creative side alive.

There is also a danger in focusing on one movement range such as running or walking. Try not to neglect other types and ranges of movement.

Everyone should always be able to squat the full range (remember the camp fire deep squat); do a push up without collapsing and sit back and then up without using their arms and keeping their legs on the floor. These movements are your birthright and will enhance the quality of your movement and therefore the quality of your life.

So are you are still with me? You are not too offended by my thoughts on the current paradigm of exercise and fitness? Good then I guess you are looking for a way of living that will bring you health, longevity, ease of movement, great mobility range and a natural level of health and fitness.

Before we get into the daily practices to start bringing your training into everyday life, I have a riddle for you: What is the best piece of exercise equipment that you are always on but never use? Turn the page for the answer.

The Floor.

The best piece of exercise equipment that we are always on, but never use.

This is a key part of the puzzle. Most programmes will have you using pieces of equipment. In many cases these are fads that get you spending your money. Much of what you encounter in the coming pages involves the use of the floor. For many it is a paradigm shift to get in touch with it again. The earth is our home. We are intimate with it as children and then as we grow, we become more and more distanced from it. A child builds its body from the ground up. It first rocks, then rolls, then crawls, cruises, falls, staggers and finally walks and runs. During this process a baby builds its body and movement patterns for life. The ground will keep you soft and relaxed in body and psyche. It will condition you and keep you able to do that all-important function of being able to get down and back up again with ease.

Movement on the ground builds and conditions your body, resets your vestibular balance and refreshes and improves your movement patterns. As mentioned above, a baby builds its body from the ground up. There is no accident in the fact that all babies go through common stages of development. Your ground movement regime can logically follow the same progression for a great ground movement session, that will leave you feeling relaxed, refreshed, connected and as tired as you want to be. Are you ready to begin? Let's try.

Stage 1: Reaching.

This is the time where a baby is starting to learn to move parts of the body independently. Believe it or not, we start to lose the ability to do this. You start by lying on your back and relaxing. Take a few deep breaths in through the nose and out through the mouth. As you exhale, relax your muscles and joints. Let your feet fall out to the side and release tension in your muscles and joints.

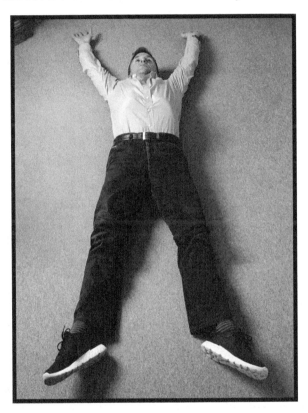

Then begin reaching with the fingers and toes gently stretching the body out in all directions. You should link your breathing and your movements. Exhale and reach, inhale and release. Gradually increase the amplitude of both the breathing and the movements. It is important ***not*** to hold the breath. Keep it flowing smoothly in and out.

Stage 2: Rolling.

Naturally then, begin rolling from the back to the front and vice versa. This process of rolling across your muscles will continue relaxing them naturally. As your muscles relax, any stress will dissolve in the body. Emotional stress is held in the body as tension. When your muscles and joints relax, stress has nothing to hold it in. As you roll, exhale. It is good to begin the rolls in the fingers and toes, like a baby would. Reach and let the reach pull you from back to front and vice versa. If you have a stiff lower back, you can also try to use the hips to roll. This is difficult, but will release your hips and back from stiffness and tension. Again exhale as you do it. This natural movement from front to back resets your vestibular balance system.

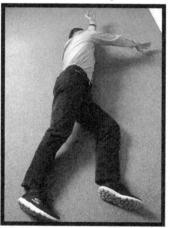

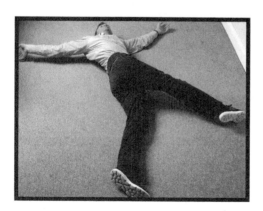

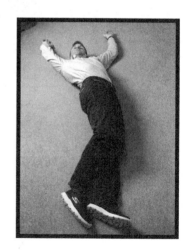

Stage 3: Time on the stomach: Time on the tummy is great as it strengthens the arms, neck and back. Use this to try pushing yourself up in a full or half (on the knees) push up. Do this softly and with smooth regular breathing.

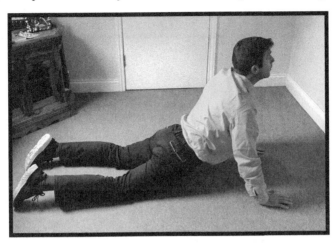

Stage 4: Sitting*:* Continuing the smooth movements from back to front now smoothly sit up and back. Try to keep the body relaxed and not tense the muscles too much. Breathe smoothly as you do it. Sit back and up again at different angles, working your oblique muscles on the side of the body. Try also to do it in a turning movement, so roll over and sit up in the same movement or inversely sit back and roll over in the same movement, so you twist the neck, shoulders, trunk and hips, checking for tension.

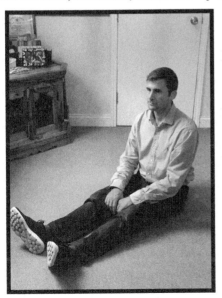
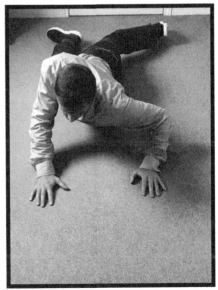

Stage 5: Crawling: A big one. Crawling is great to test your muscles, joints, cardio-vascular system, bilateral coordination and to reset your vestibular system.

Begin by leopard crawling, forwards and backwards

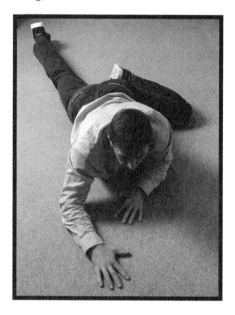

Then transition to your back moving with the feet and shoulders.

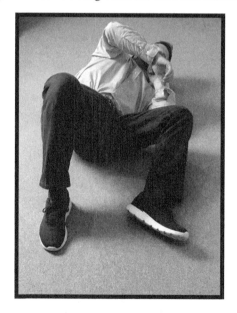

Then transition to baby crawl on your hands and knees.

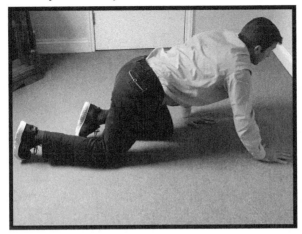

Then begin to increase the amplitude of the movement as in the picture below.

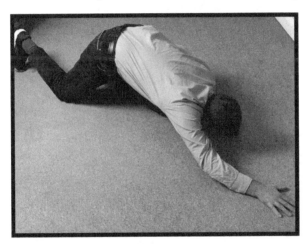

Important:

Make sure that you move opposite hand and foot at the same time so that you train in the right motor skills and movement patterns. I have noticed when I teach in schools, that children who have coordination problems also have problems doing this movement. It is also interesting to note that their parents often say that they didn't crawl as children. However, it is also my experience that these children and even adults can remedy these coordination problems by going back and spending time correcting the ability to crawl, using the right movement pattern of opposite hand and foot moving at the same time.

You should also try this going sideways:

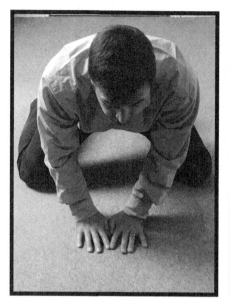 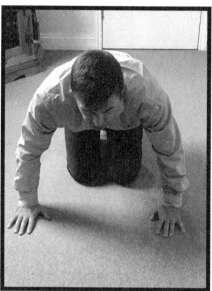

Then try it backwards. When going backwards look over the shoulder as per the picture below.

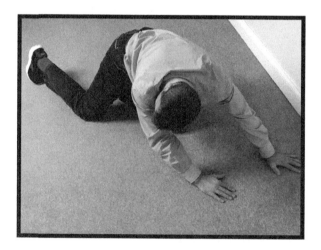

This gives a good stretch in the neck and works all the muscles down your side. As with many movements, it is important to try them going forwards, backwards and sideways. Try your movements through all directions and angles.

Important: To have rounded movement we need to go backwards. We spend most of our life in a forward position. Driving, walking, working, watching screens, sitting etc. are all forward movements. It is important for balance in your muscles, movements and psyche to also practice movements backwards.

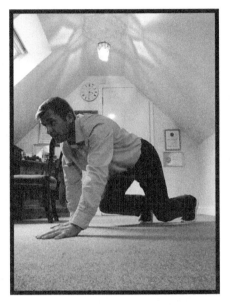

Then try an elevated baby crawl. This is sometimes referred to as the Spiderman crawl. Simply raise the knees a couple of inches off the floor (see picture below) and do the same movement.

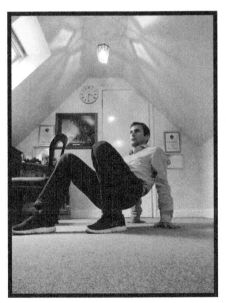

This will put more stress through the joints and muscles working them and giving you more of a cardio vascular test. It is important to maintain the opposite hand and foot pattern in the movement.
Also try this in a crab position as in the picture below.

Again it is important to move opposite hand opposite foot. For most people this will be more difficult than the baby crawl.

Tip: If you struggle with the transition from knees down to knees elevated, try it going up and down the stairs in your home for a week. Every time you come up or down the stairs go up forwards and down backwards. You will accomplish this before you know it.

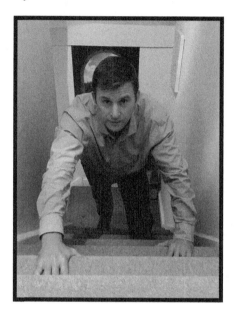

An advanced level of the crawl is to try it on a plank, log or beam. The narrowed nature of this will check your stabilising muscles much more.

Challenge exercise: Try to crawl continuously for 10 minutes in the crab or Spiderman crawl. It will be very important to breathe correctly; otherwise you will become tired very quickly. Inhale one movement, exhale one movement. If this is too difficult, try to increase by 90 seconds each day for one week.

Crawling will also improve your reflexive strength or reflexive stability. This makes you more resilient, stable and mobile.

Stage 6: Standing and falling. A good skill to develop is falling softly. This was covered in my previous book (Systema Health: 25 practices for a lifetime of health, fitness and wellbeing). This is such an important skill that I have included it here for those who don't have that book.

The ground is hard. Even if carpeted. This will keep you soft and relaxed.

There are many people over middle age in western culture who, if you asked them to get down to the floor and up again, would struggle. The reason for the struggle is that their bodies are too stiff. Their joints won't bend enough to avoid collapsing with a bump. They also do the movement with fear and trepidation of hurting themselves. Older people are terrified of falling. This fear itself causes them to be brittle. Many older people in western cultures don't recover from falls. It remains the biggest cause of death in old age. Contrast this to a toddler, who is constantly falling, rolling or diving to the floor and getting back up again. There is no fear and rarely do they damage themselves. To be able to get to the floor smoothly and back up again without fear of injury or actual injury is a life skill. Especially when it is an unexpected fall. So how do you do it? Well there is no set technique, but there are principles. They are as follows:

1. Do it softly. There should be no noise or bumps. Just a soft exhale.
2. Go down on your muscles not bones. Keep the elbows, knees, fingers and wrists safe.
3. Try to be like a soft ball, not a 50 pence piece (pentagon shape).
4. Breathe out as you go down to the ground.
5. Roll out the impact of the fall.

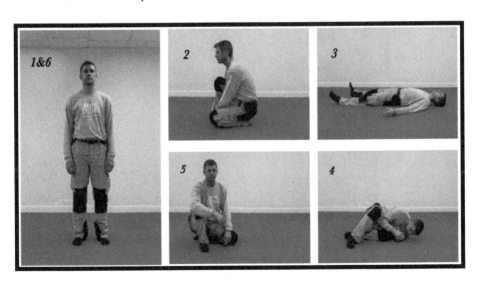

The floor is your base. Build from here. It is a great teacher. One that will keep you moving smoothly and easily well into old age.

The next chapter begins the main emphasis of the book. It gives 20 simple ways to begin integrating training into your everyday life. 20 ways to live Systema.

Bringing Systema Into Everyday Life.

20 everyday moments to train and live Systema.

What follows are 20 ways to bring healthy, relaxed, free movement back into your body. In everyday moments. A system that is not a dogmatic. A regimen that makes existence your training. One that will give you a level of health and physicality that is way above average, that is sustainable for a lifetime and affords you a quality of movement and therefore a quality of life that is your birthright.

It is about making the seconds count. Being conscious of every second, because we don't fall apart or decay overnight. You have to be mindful and pay attention to every second. Why? Because seconds lead to minutes, to hours, days and suddenly years of bad habits have gone by. How do we pay attention to the seconds or moments? By paying attention to the small things and doing them right.

Of course this is not limited to 20. These are examples. You can and should evolve, adapt and add to these. You have to make them yours. This is a key concept of Systema that separates it from many other arts. It is not about learning someone else's techniques. You have to own it. You embody the principles and then allow them to seep from your very pores into everything that you do.

I have broken the 20 activities out into four categories:

The physical set

1. 1-1 Strength – Your basic requirements.
2. Look no hands.
3. Squat don't bend.
4. Sit on your bones.
5. Daily constitutional: Walk as you were born to.
6. Get down!
7. The 10 natural sitting positions challenge.
8. Posture Checks.
9. Elbows off the table.
10. Stair Crawls.

The breathing set

11. Release with your breath.
12. Cold shower burst breathing.
13. Breathe then move.

The balance set

14. Stand on one leg while brushing your teeth.
15. Do as much as you can with your feet.
16. Put your shoes and socks on while standing up.

The tension set

17. Tension awareness.
18. Tension and relaxation before sleep.
19. Continual small adjustments.

Final Note

20. Cultivate a playful attitude.

1. 1-1 Strength – your basic requirements.

Ok so the first one is not a moment, it is a foundation. One that needs to become a 'maintenance moment'. But this is so important that it has to be number one. You need to get to a stage where these four movements are effortless. This may take weeks, months or years. It doesn't matter. Each day will bring you improvements. It is not a destination, it is a continuum. 1:1 strength, or put another way, the ability to move your body smoothly through its natural range of movements without compensation, is a great indicator of your overall level of health. If you can't, it means that you are either too heavy for your strength, or too weak for your weight. This should not only be slightly embarrassing (sorry to be harsh here) but it is also impinging the quality of your life and probably the length of it to.

The tests:

You should be able to smoothly and easily do these 5 movements.
- Laying on your tummy push your body up in one straight piece (i.e. not using knees) and lower yourself in one straight piece under control.
- Standing upright, lower yourself using only your legs to a deep squat position, then return smoothly back to standing without using your arms on your legs.
- From a seated floor position sit back flat and then return to a seated position, without using the hands and keeping your heels on the floor.
- From a supine position (laying on your back) lift the legs up to horizontal (go right over if you can and touch the floor with your toes) then lower again, keeping the lumber (lower) area of your back and your head flat on the floor.

- From a brachial (overhand) dead hang (arms straight muscles relaxed), smoothly pull your chin over a bar or branch and then lower under control.

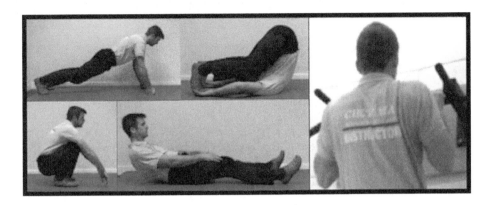

None of these movements are Olympic level or even particularly athletic. If you think about it they are a starting point.

I know that the pull up is tough, especially an overhand grasp, but it is a life-saving skill too. Consider pulling yourself out of the window of a burning building, or out of a shear sided in soaking wet clothes bank after falling in water, or back over a cliff edge etc. You probably won't be using an underhand grasp for this.

If you can do some of these, but not others, then you are imbalanced. It is worth correcting this imbalance. Your body is intricately connected. Weakness in one area affects others (think weak or tight hamstrings and lower back problems).

If you can do these movements your quality of life will soar. We are living a physical existence. We are not (yet) Mekons i.e. big brains moved around on a weak and puny body. Limitation in our body is limitation in our experience of life. The freedom to play, to run, jump, roll, crawl, climb, swing on a rope, have fun and fully engage in all the activities that life has to offer. If your body is in pain, you really can't concentrate on much else.

Notice that I did not use the term, 'exercises' once. These are **natural movements**. Your birthright. They should be do-able and with you right to the end. You should not need to set aside time to do them, they should be part of your everyday life. There is no need to age badly. You should be able to get yourself up and down stairs without a Stannah Stair lift and in and out of the bath unaided, whatever your age. The rot sets in early, when we stop moving fully and regularly.

If you struggle with this don't be disheartened. It is reversible. Whatever your age. Just patiently and diligently do these 1:1 strength movements once per day, as slowly as you can.

To view the free video of this practise please use the link below: http://www.matthill.co.uk/living-systema

2. Look no hands.

In many ways our hands are cheats instead of using our bodies correctly. We incorrectly use them for everyday actions like lowering into a chair, holding a handrail walking down or up stairs, getting into and out of a car (not the opening the door part), lowering and pulling ourselves up when putting something away in a low cupboard etc. One of the biggest is putting our hands on our knees to push up as we stand. Most people use the hands to aid themselves in these tasks. When you do this, the work of the legs and the core are seriously impaired.

Whenever you do any of these movements, try to do so without using the hands. This will mean that you squat with the legs taking the full load of the body. As you adjust your position in the chair, again avoid using the hands. This will mean using your core muscles to manouever yourself.

Add 100 squats to your day. Every day.
Now of course this is not like a gym workout. However it is a little, a lot. Think of the amount of times you sit and then stand again. How many times do you do it in a day? Depending on your job, I would say at least 100. Think about it. Getting out of bed, getting breakfast out of a low cupboard, sitting for breakfast, getting up, getting into your car or onto transport, getting out, sitting at your desk. Then, when you are at your desk, how many times a day do you get up and down? At least three times an hour I'm guessing. If you don't then you should. So that is six squats per hour. For 8 hours of the day. Then reverse that process getting home. Add in a few miscellaneous ones and you have between 70 and 100 squats per day.

Tips to make the movement better.

Sitting. Approach the chair backwards with it behind you. Touch the chair with your calves, plant the feet firmly and sit smoothly and lightly. See picture below:

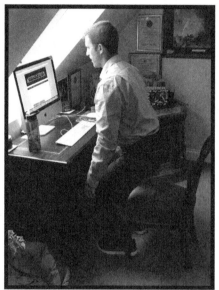

Standing. Shuffle forwards without the use of the hands until your feet are planted fully on the floor. Then stand smoothly, in one fluid movement with no rocking or momentum and of course without using the hands.

Bonus points: As you progress, or if you are already at a decent stage, try to incorporate these types of sits too.

Recliner or sofa: When you sit on a recliner or sofa, especially with elevated feet, the same rules apply. Don't pull yourself forwards with your hands. Sit yourself up using only your stomach muscles and core, shuffle forwards and then stand.

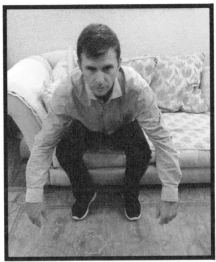

Car: Try to get in and out of your car without using your hands. This is trickier, but try to smoothly slide in and out, without momentum. Your agility, core and leg strength, balance and confidence will begin to improve very quickly. If you have a driving job, this is a great tip.

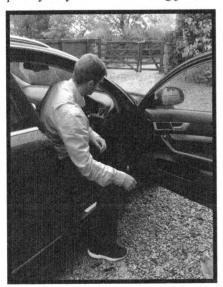 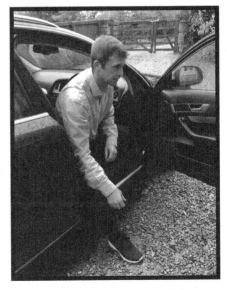

To view the free video of this practise please use the link below:
http://www.matthill.co.uk/living-systema

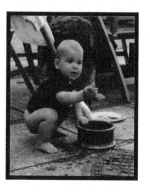

Squat Don't Bend.

When you watch someone in counties like the Middle and Far East, India and Africa bend down to pick something up, what do you see? I guarantee it will either be the natural deep squat, or straight leg, straight back bend if they are working in the field. This one is fine too of course, the key is a straight back. Squatting rather than bending is a great way to get more of the regular benefits of squatting, which include but are not limited to:

- Injury prevention (stops you straining and bending the lower back)
- Ease of everyday movement (getting up and down is probably the most common movement and the one that people struggle with most as they get older)
- Power generation (for martial artists or athletes most power, balance and movement comes from a squat)
- Softness in the legs for balance and smoothness. This is a big one. By focusing on exhaling and relaxing EVERY time you squat (bend) you will keep your legs supple by removing tension.
- Improved digestion and bowel movement. Another big one. By doing a correct squat (often called the baby or toilet squat) you will massage your colon and improve your digestion and bowel movements the way nature intended.
- Improved vasal and lymphatic circulation.
- Improved viscera function.

This is the way you were born to move. Watch a baby when they lower themselves to play or pick something up. They certainly don't copy the example of their parents or brothers and sisters in the western world.

So the challenge here is that whenever you reach down to pick something up, get something off the lower shelf of a supermarket, put the washing in the machine, empty the dishwasher or pick your socks up off the floor, *squat, don't bend.*

If you do keep the legs straight and bend from the waist, make sure that it is a straight leg, straight back bend as you see when you see people working the rice fields as per the picture below. This way you still get the benefit of maintaining good posture.

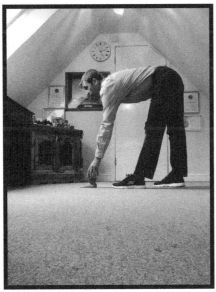

To view the free video of this practise please use the link below: http://www.matthill.co.uk/living-systema

4. Sit on your bones.

Most people in the western world spend an average of 14 hours per day sat on their backsides.

I know that for some people there is no other option: drivers, office workers etc.

There is however, a great way to manage this.

When you sit, you can alleviate a lot of the poor postural problems by sitting on your sitting bones. See picture below:

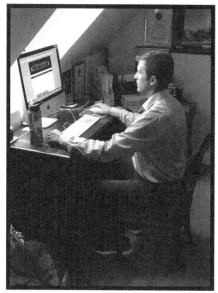

Good Posture.

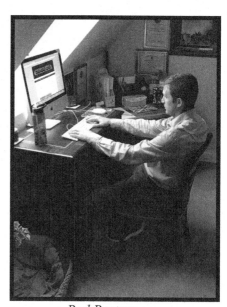

Bad Posture.

Sitting in bad posture has several problems:

1. It allows you to sit for a long time, and sitting for a long time is not good for us. Our bodies need and benefit from movement. Almost constantly. We are not designed to spend much more than 20 minutes in one position before changing. On page 33 you will find the, '10 natural sitting positions challenge'. You will find that you cannot hold these positions for long without wanting to change position. This will become apparent when you try Practise 7, *The 10 Natural Sitting Positions*, on page 34.

2. As a martial artist you should always be ready to move to safety in one smooth movement. If you have to first sit up straight, then adjust the feet and then stand and move that will be too late. If you are sitting on the bones of your bum you will be able to stand in one fluid movement.

3. When you sit in bad posture you will be putting pressure in the wrong areas of your body. Gravity will be pushing your weight out of the area where your posture is kinked, or weak. This could be your lower back, sternum, neck or a number of other places. Over time this will cause a problem. In the short term you will be stiff in that area and in the long term you are likely to develop structural or tension related issues.

To remedy this, as you sit you should feel your two pelvic bones, one on either side. If you can't feel them say on a cushioned chair, try sitting on a hard chair or the floor.

As long as you can feel these bones, your posture is good. Feet should be planted flat underneath you.

Point 2 (above) is an important point to note about posture. For much of our existence on the planet we didn't know what was going to happen next. We could be attacked at any moment from behind a bush or rock. Today as a martial artist you train for the time when you don't know what is going to happen next, such as an imminent attack. This could come as you are sat or stood on the bus, train, tube, wherever. In this instance your posture would be more neutral – ready to move any part of you in any direction, freely and spontaneously.

As soon as you slouch backwards (see picture above) you will become kyphotic in your posture, causing the problems outlined above.

So there are two good checks:
1. Can you feel the bones of your bum?
2. Can you stand in one fluid movement?

If you can answer yes to both of these then your posture is fine.

If not, reconsider it.

Key point:

It is hard to maintain this for any length of time. 10-20 minutes is about average. Funnily enough this is also the length of time after which it is suggested that we stand and walk for a few minutes if sat down. So this can be your alarm clock if you spend a lot of time at a desk. As soon as you feel yourself come off the bones of your bum, stand up, reset, get a drink of water and then sit down again. This will also have the added benefit of resting your eyes, shoulders, arms and wrists.

To view the free video of this practise please use the link below:
http://www.matthill.co.uk/living-systema

5. The daily constitutional.
Walk as you were born to.

When I first talk about relearning your walk at Systema classes I can see people looking at me dubiously. After all, they have been walking ok for their whole lives.

The difference is that I want them to walk in a way that promotes health, not just in terms of calorie burn, but also in terms of resetting the system and removing stress.

Walking is the defining movement of a human being and the great thing about walking is that you can't be sitting at the same time.

Few people in the western world walk enough. In Victorian times it was called the daily constitutional. We knew just how good and vital it was for the optimum functioning of our body and system. The benefits are well documented:

- Calorie burn.
- Endorphin release (mood enhancers).
- Toning of the muscles.
- Strengthening of the heart.
- Reduction in risk of diseases such as diabetes and cancer.
- Fresh air (when taken in a natural environment).

This is all good. With a little bit of added knowledge however, you can get much more bang for your buck.

Walking is our natural reset button. It is how we calm ourselves down, relax and unwind. We know this intuitively. Take for example when someone is stressed or angry. We will find ourselves saying to them, "Come on let's go for a walk." Within a few minutes of walking they will start to calm down, breathe deeply and the stress will begin to melt away.

Adding just a few elements to improve your walking can enhance the effects stated above. Daily life puts stress in our bodies:
- Physical stress from sitting too much, or from physical work in a poor position, such as digging.
- Stress from bad sitting posture, as highlighted in the previous chapter.
- Emotional stress of deadlines, workloads, financial problems etc.

The emotional stresses begin as a thought or worry and quickly become physical tension in the body. We often slump as if under the weight of the problem. Shoulders become hunched, brown furrowed, head hanging forward, chest kyphosis etc.

Walking is our natural antidote to this. When walking correctly you literally breathe and walk the stress out of your body.

Here are a few steps to help this.
1) *Focus on your breathing*. Try to link it to your steps. This is called the *Russian Breath Ladder*. Breathe in through your nose for say 4 steps and then out through your mouth for 4 steps. If this is too difficult try one, two or three and then build up. As you relax and improve you can stretch this to 6, 8, 10 or more. You then also get all the benefits of nasal breathing that I have outlined in previous books and blogs. (These benefits are also included as an annex at the end of the book along with details of how to do the Russian Breath Ladder. Turn to Annex 3 to read them if you are not sure.)
2) *Relax on the exhale*. As you exhale, try to relax your muscles from the head down to the feet. You can do this over a number of breaths. So on the first breath, as you inhale, bring your attention to your face and head, then as you exhale relax that area. On the second breath as you inhale bring your attention to your neck, as you exhale relax it. You can do more than one breath for each body part; do as many as you need. Then proceed to go right through the body. A suggestion for the order is below:

- Face and head.
- Neck.
- Shoulders.
- Arms.
- Chest and upper back.
- Sternum and middle back.
- Stomach and lower back.
- Hips and glutes.
- Thighs and hamstrings.
- Knees.
- Calves and shins.
- Ankles.
- Feet.

Then finish with complete breaths that begin at the top and fall right through the body to the feet. So breathe in and become aware of your whole body. Then exhale and be aware of each part as you relax down through the whole body.

3) *Walk from the knees*. To do this, begin your step by relaxing and moving the knee forwards. This sounds strange but it is the way we are designed to walk. Not with stiff stilt like legs, but in a relaxed smooth fluid movement beginning in the knees. This will relax your leg muscles, make you more energy efficient, lighten your step reducing impact and make you more balanced over uneven terrain.

4) *Maintain a good posture*. An important point to note is that this is **not** like a military recruit posture that has too much tension. Begin at the top. Your chin should be gently pulled in but not up. Make sure there is no tension in your neck as you do this. Your chest should be lifted slightly and gently pulled out. Your back muscles should be relaxed. This will relax your shoulders and arms into their natural position. They should be loose and relaxed at your sides. This will ensure that you are not building tension, pain or future problems through bad posture.

5) *Try to neutralise your posture*. Try not to have a sway or swagger in your walk. It should be fluid and neutral. A sway, strut or swagger in your walk is a waste of energy and will also make you stand out. There may well be times when you do not want to stand out. I am sure that you can think of

some. It is good to practice how to move in a way that you are seen but not noticed. Nothing about your normal walk should attract attention. When you can neutralize your walk you have normalized it. From this base, it is then easy to add things to your walk should you wish.

Your body should feel light; In fact, your body should 'disappear' to your senses. The only time you should feel your posture, is if you are in pain or tense. If you are relaxed, injury free and in good posture you should not feel your body. All you should feel is the contact of your feet on the floor.

It obviously helps to walk outside in fresh air, preferably in proximity to trees. When you walk with these five points in mind you will amplify the benefit of getting outside and dosing up on vitamin D.

Sometimes we are very much like a computer that has had to process too much. We need to hit the reset button. Our natural reset is walking. Even a very short walk of say a few minutes is enough if we are keeping these points in mind. In fact as I write this, the National Health Service in the UK (NHS) is promoting 'Active 10'. This is an initiative to get people doing 10 minutes of brisk walking per day to improve all round health and wellbeing.

Walking is the form of exercise that has the lowest drop out rate. Combining daily walking, ideally 3-5 miles per day, with a healthy diet of all round movement is probably the best medicine you can give to your body.

I know that many people struggle to find time to walk, especially those with office jobs. Here are some ideas:
- During your lunch break, go for a walk.
- Use the stairs instead of the lift.
- Walk to speak to colleagues rather than (or as well as) sending them emails. Walk around the house if you are taking calls on the phone.
- Do walking meetings and calls.
- Where practical park your car as far as possible away from your location and then walk to work or your destination.
- Get out of the bus/underground a stop earlier and walk the extra mile.

- Get a dog (but only if you will walk it regularly and love it!)
- Make everyday activities walks – shopping, meeting a friend, dates, date nights, returning calls, brainstorming or planning etc.
- Walk as a family and then combine it with playing: hide and seek, tag, off ground tag etc.
- If you do have an office job where you sit most of the day, the best thing you can do is to get a standing desk at work, or just put your computer on a box that will put it at the right height for you to stand up.

To view the free video of this practise please use the link below: http://www.matthill.co.uk/living-systema

6. Get down!

At least once per day.

Use it or lose it. This is another simple one. AT LEAST once per day, make sure that you sit on the floor. Whether it is to play with a pet, a child or grandchild, whilst watching TV, or any other of a number of reasons. Some of you may have jobs which require you to get down a lot, e.g. plumbers, electricians etc. If that is the case, great. Now you just need to focus on doing this action in a way that will promote health and relaxation in the body and not damage it over time.

It is important that you don't become a stranger to the act of getting down to the floor and back up again with ease. If you do, there will eventually come a time in your life when you can't do it. There is no reason for this to happen. This action should be available to us right to the end.

There is also another important reason. As we age, falling becomes a very real fear for people. As I mentioned earlier in the book, statistically falls are the biggest killer in old age. When people fall they often never recover. Those that do are terrified of falling again. This fear makes them very anxious, stiff and brittle and causes further mobility problems.

When they are on the floor, many don't have the mobility, confidence or strength to get up again, especially if there is nothing to hold onto to pull them up. This is a problem with using the hands too much for everyday things (see practise 1: Look no hands). Their muscles and balance will be weak or non-existent in the low range and so standing from the floor without help will be very difficult, especially when in shock or pain. This is a very modern problem. A person who regularly (as in several times per day) puts their body through that action of getting to the ground and up again, with ease and smoothness will have no fear of falling. It is also important to put your psyche through this action daily so that it is not unfamiliar. People that do this regularly will then have no problem standing up again, even if injured.

Key points:
1. Exhale first then lower yourself. DON'T hold your breath in the process of getting down or up.
2. Try to limit the amount that you use your hands for support. This way you will use your legs and core much more effectively. It will also improve your balance and stability. Additionally if you injure yourself in a fall, it improves your ability to get back up with a broken arm or wrist.
3. Try to be as smooth as possible in the movement. Do it slowly and notice any holding of the breath or tension in your muscles that is not needed (especially shoulders) and strain on your joints. You are aiming for the body to remain soft, balanced and even.

For many this (without the use of hands) is a hard thing to do. Try it bit by bit. Think of the following scale when it comes to this or any other activity or movement:

Strive to make the impossible possible, the hard easy and the easy elegant. - Moshe Feldenkrais.

Elegant here means effortless and completely in balance the whole time when it comes to this movement.

To view the free video of this practise please use the link below: http://www.matthill.co.uk/living-systema

7. The 10 Natural sitting positions challenge.

This section is linked closely to the previous section. Before the advent of chairs, most of our time would have been spent on the floor. In fact sitting is being framed as the smoking of this generation, in terms of the damage that it is doing to our health. Experts say that you can't smoke cigarettes fast enough to replicate the damage that prolonged sitting does.

Sitting weakens our hamstrings and core muscles, hunches our shoulders, and gives us a kyphotic posture. Chairs are far too comfortable, allowing us to stay static in one position far longer than we ever could. This comfort is killing us softly. There are some scary statistics attached to it.

It increases cancer by 10%, heart disease by 6% and Type 2 diabetes by 7%. It also has a dramatic effect on our mobility. It cuts our natural squat range in half (see pictures below):

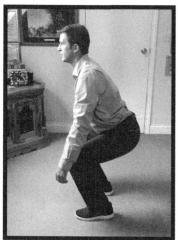 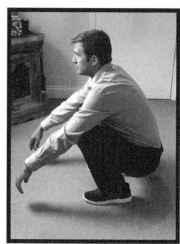

The problem is that we don't question it. Everyone else is doing it too. Everywhere. The average person in the western world now spends 9.3 hours sitting down. Many will spend significantly more than that. If you didn't clock it in the sitting positions practise, I will reiterate it here. The best thing that you can do if you have a sitting office job is to get a standing workstation. Failing that, a box that you put your computer on that enables you to stand and work.

The ten positions outlined below, were our way of sitting or resting before the advent of chairs. They are the way to begin reversing the damage that prolonged sitting is doing to our bodies. They will be hard at first but they will bring youthful movement back to your body. They will start to turn the clock back and reverse the degenerative process in your body.

In all probability, the last time that you will have attempted some of these positions was when you were a child. They are a great way to check:
- Leg, hip and lower back strength.
- Suppleness.
- Stability.
- Balance.
- Longevity.

The Challenge:
1. Try each of the 10 positions.
2. Where appropriate try them on your left side and right side.
3. Check how comfortable they are. You should be able to sit for at least 10 minutes in each of them.
4. Make getting down and back up smoothly and effortlessly a requirement. Try not to use your hands or elbows to assist. For bonus points, try not to use your knees either. This is deceptively tricky.

The pictures below show all 10 positions. There is also a video that can be obtained here: https://www.youtube.com/watch?v=OY4dQx2oSrU. Barring injury, they should be attainable for us all.

There will come a time when, if we are not doing this regularly, you will not be able to get to the floor and back up. We all want this ability in our bodies right to the end.

So to keep youthful movement in your body, try to start spending more time sat on the floor, playing with children, with pets, watching TV whatever. Then when you stand, move smoothly, exhale as you move, and try not to use your hands.

You will reap the rewards of this very quickly. Good luck and let me know how you do!

The 10 Positions

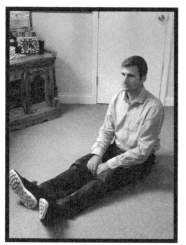

Straight leg sit

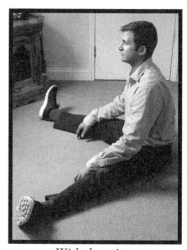

Wide leg sit

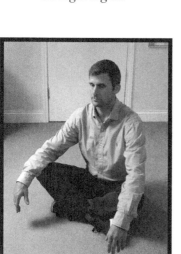

Cross leg sit

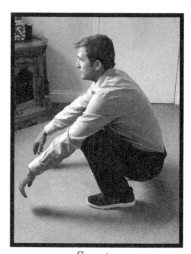

Squat

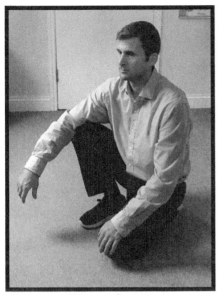

Hunter Squat

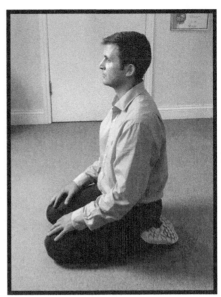

Kneeling

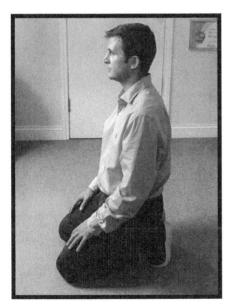

Kneeling toes up

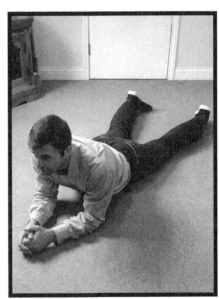

Lying prone

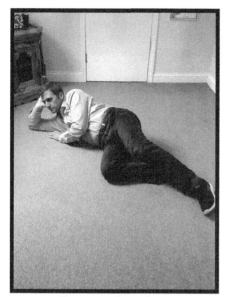 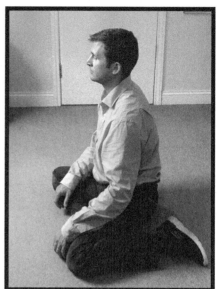

Lying on the side   *Z-sit*

To view the free video of this practise please use the link below:
http://www.matthill.co.uk/living-systema

8. Posture Checks.

We all carry around far more tension in our body than is needed. This practise is a great way to start noticing this tension during everyday activities such as making a cup of tea (very British I know), standing in a queue (also very British I know), watching a sports match or any other time that you are standing for a period of time.

Use those moments when you are engaged in this kind of activity to exhale and relax your muscles. You will be amazed at how tense your shoulders, arms, neck, hips and legs etc. are. You want your muscles to be relaxed and hanging loosely off the bones like water balloons. Often we are the opposite, we are holding our body up with tension, like air balloons.

Tips for good posture:
- Eyes are looking straight ahead with neck muscles relaxed. Your head should have some 'play' in it like a gear stick in neutral.
- Chin is pulled in slightly but not so much that it tenses the neck.
- Chest is opened up and out but not so much that it tenses the muscles in the back.
- Arms 'hang' neutrally at the sides in their natural position.
- Hips 'hang' neutrally.
- Knees are relaxed and just slightly bent, but not so much that the leg muscles are tense.

Strive to have only the amount of muscular effort in the body that it requires to do the work that it is doing, i.e. standing. See picture below:

You have three great tools to help you do this:

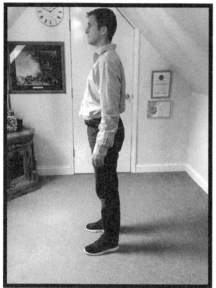

1. Breathing. Use your breathing like a scan. As you inhale feel for any tension in your body. Much like blowing up a balloon. Imagine trying to inflate a balloon, which has some areas of the material that are stiffer than others. These areas will be harder to inflate. When you find them, try to release them first with an exhale. If the exhale doesn't work try:
2. Movement. Subtle shifts and movements in the body will let you know which areas are tense, allowing you to let go of them with an exhale.
3. Tension and relaxation. If you have trouble letting the tension go, try to tense the area on an inhale and then relax it again as you exhale.

A natural posture will be efficient muscularly. Poor posture will add tension to your body in the areas of bad posture and will also refer tension to other areas. A straight body posture will relax you. Good posture literally allows tension to fall out of the body into the ground.

This will help you to conserve energy, improve circulation and avoid chronic muscle strain and fatigue over time.

To view the free video of this practise please use the link below:
http://www.matthill.co.uk/living-systema

9. Elbows off the table.

Do you ever remember your parents telling you to get your elbows off the table?

It wasn't just about good manners. It's about good digestion and building good core strength and posture in the everyday things. At a deeper level it is also about maintaining a positive outlook and making a good impression.

We spend so much time sitting and eating that it would be a real shame not to make the most of these opportunities.

Good posture when eating helps the food go down better. A straight body rather than a slouched body aids the digestive process.

As well as being told at home not to put my elbows on the table, I was told the same thing during my time in Japan. In Japan they took it a step further. When eating food out of a bowl, they would bring the bowl to their mouths to either sip or eat, in order to avoid any bending of the body.

As well as the dinner table you should also try to do this at work. If you have a desk job try to avoid using chairs with an armrest. Same thing when in a car. It will also help you to stay much more alert while driving, or if you are in a long meeting on a hot day. Two times when you really don't want to be feeling drowsy!

The same principle can be extended to waiting while standing. Try not to lean against a wall or a post, but rather stand relaxed and at ease in good posture.

You then more naturally adopt the same principle as outlined in practise 4: Sit on the bones of your bum.

To view the free video of this practise please use the link below: http://www.matthill.co.uk/living-systema

10. Stair Crawls.

In the process of building the body from the ground up as outlined in the practise on floor work, the importance of the crawl was discussed.

Lots of people have trouble with this at the start. The trouble usually comes in four forms:

1. The strength in the muscles to support the weight.
2. The strength or flexibility in the joints to support the weight.
3. The ability to coordinate opposite hand and opposite leg, moving at the same time, in the way that we do while standing.
4. The cardio vascular ability to keep going past a minute or two.

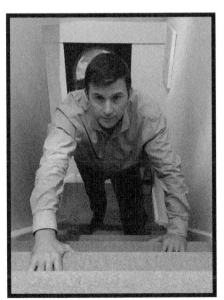

A good way to overcome these problem areas is do them on an incline. The stairs in your house are a good time to practise. Equally a hill is good too if you are out on a walk.

The work is simple. When you ascend put your hands down and go up the stairs in an elevated crawl or Spiderman crawl.

As you descend, come down backwards again in Spiderman crawl. It is important to still maintain the habit of good breaths; inhale one movement, exhale one movement. As you improve you can extend that to inhale two movements exhale two movements, then three, then four etc. See how far up the breath ladder you can go with this.

After a short period of doing this, all four elements of your crawl will improve. Your general cardio vascular level will improve. Your all over strength will improve (these exercises target a lot of muscles). Your all round hand eye coordination will improve, as you improve the motor skill of opposite hand opposite foot movements. The health and functionality of your joints will also improve.

Advanced exercise:

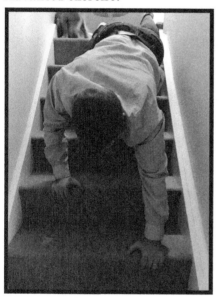

To increase your strength and confidence in this exercise, you can try going up the stairs facing downwards and coming back down the stairs also facing downwards.

This takes a lot more strength and will test you more in all four areas. It may be better to try this on a hill first where you have a soft landing if you slip.

To view the free video of this practise please use the link below: http://www.matthill.co.uk/living-systema

The breathing set.

The following three practises are ways to consciously bring the Systema breathing method into your training. Correct breathing is a central pillar of Systema. Without a deep understanding of the breathing, nothing else will work to your full potential. For those readers who are new to Systema, it is better to have a basic understanding of Systema breathing as outlined below.

My first book, Systema health: '*25 Practices For A Lifetime Of Health, Fitness And Wellbeing*', has a comprehensive chapter on breathing.

You can also get the corresponding video on Pivotshare: (https://matthill.pivotshare.com/authors/matt-hill/7720/media), or just Google: 'Matt Hill Pivotshare'.

The basics of Systema breathing are simple:

- You breathe in through the nose,
- Out through the mouth and;
- Make it continuous.

This last point about making it continuous sounds ridiculously obvious and simple I know. However, you all hold your breath far more than you are aware. The most common response I get when people start Systema is, "wow, I never realised how much I hold my breath!"

Why is this bad?

There are many things that can make us hold our breath:

- When we are emotionally affected by anxiety, fear, panic or shock.
- When doing physical movements, even standing up from a chair for example.
- When our mind gets distracted by something e.g. a beautiful sunrise, or a beautiful person walking past. They literally 'take our breath away'.
- Pain.
- When we concentrate hard.

When we stop breathing, restrictive tension floods into the body, our ability to think widely and creatively diminishes; our ability to endure falls off a cliff (if we are in a combat mode we will 'gas' or become exhausted very quickly.) and our movements and thinking become erratic and panicky.

The final point is that we need to adjust the speed of breathing to the demands of the situation. I.e. the greater the pressure, the faster the breathing. So when everything is normal and calm, a smooth, long, light breath is the best. It should be virtually inaudible and devoid of tension. As the pressure increases, be it physical, mental or emotional, so should the rate of breathing. This may happen gradually as in a gentle transition in speed or pace of walking or running, or it may happen in a heartbeat such as a sudden stab of pain, injury, attack or shock. In Systema we call this 'burst breathing.' It is rather like a sound of a steam train, but still needs to be in through the nose and out through the mouth. The burst breathing continues for as long as needed and then gradually returns to long, smooth, calm breaths. This can be accompanied by subtle movements of the body, especially the shoulders, arms, hips and legs, to check for and then release tension.

To view the free video of this practise please use the link below: http://www.matthill.co.uk/living-systema

11. Release with your breath.

As explained in the previous practice, we generally hold our breath when something bothers us. This practise is about becoming more mindful and more embodied.

You need to first notice this and then decompress yourself with a relaxing exhale.

The exhale is much like an old fashioned pressure cooker. Holding your breath will build pressure fast, exhaling will release that pressure.

The exhale should be relaxed. Like a sigh. No tension in the chest, abdomen, throat, or cheeks. The mouth should be relaxed not pinched and you exhale from the lips in a 'puh' sound. Try not to blow out with a pinched 'o' shape to the mouth, with a 'huh' sound from the chest, or with a constricted sound from the throat.

Holding your breath, even for a short time, will have the following effects: It will diminish your performance and lock the body up by:

- Tensing the muscles,
- Heightening anxiety,
- Increasing heart rate and blood pressure,
- Diminishing thinking capacity and creative open thinking in high stress situations,
- Freezing you in position.

So this exercise is simple. Become more aware of your breathing on a moment-to-moment basis. As soon as you notice that you have stopped breathing, even for a few seconds, exhale and the restore to normal relaxed breaths.

To view the free video of this practise please use the link below: http://www.matthill.co.uk/living-systema

12. Cold Shower Burst breathing.

This one is great for hitting several areas. It is cold immersion training; strengthens your will, breath training and just plain healthy.

The benefits of cold-water immersion have been espoused by many people from Florence Nightingale to Henry David Thoreau. Its many benefits include:

- Strengthening the immune system.
- Helping weight loss.
- Relaxation.
- Helping with stress and depression.
- Increasing circulation.
- Increases alertness.
- Lowering blood pressure and heart rate.

All of these are great. The reason that I have included it however, *is to practise burst breathing.*

Burst breathing is used when we don't have access to long, smooth, calm breaths. Examples are:

- Physical exertion.
- When we are in pain, fear or panic or,
- When you jump into a cold river, lake or just taking a cold shower.

To do the burst breath you do a quick exhale through the mouth followed by an immediate inhale. The inhale is literally a sniff. The exhale is a short puff making a 'puh' sound with the mouth as described in Practise 11.

During times of high pressure we need a bridging breath. This, bridging or, 'burst' breath will allow you to keep breathing through the difficult time and then relax back to long, calm relaxed breaths.

So, wash first in warm or hot water. Then when you have finished, switch your shower to cold and try to do 100 burst breaths. You can of course build to this. So try with 10 first, then 20 next time, then 30 etc. Keep building until you can do 100. Once you can get to 100, much more should be do-able.

It will be a shock at first; you manage the shock with a focus on your burst breathing. The rapid repetition of the breaths will assist you in staying focused and managing the cold. As you progress it will get easier and easier.

Remember that cold showers are great, but if you can, get out to a river, a lake, the sea, a waterfall or even use a bucket of cold water left outside overnight.

To view the free video of this practise please use the link below: http://www.matthill.co.uk/living-systema

13. Breathe then move.

Breathwork is the key to Systema and of course life. We don't get far without it. Most of us however, hold our breath a lot throughout the day. Especially when we move.

You will have noticed it with the four pillars of Systema (Practise 1). If you don't know what these are, they are explained in depth in the Systema Health book. When the body is under physical strain, most people hold their breath. Starting today, try to consciously exhale when you move. For example when you sit down or stand up in a chair, begin your exhale THEN move.

At a slightly more advanced level you can exhale as you sit, and as you stand inhale. In a way, this is more natural. As you sit you compress and deflate the body a little. This motion would naturally release the air. Then as you stand you naturally inflate the body with an inhale. You are also then ready for your next movement after standing.

I have used a sit and stand as an example as it is a very common movement throughout the day. It can and should of course be used with every movement. Bending, lifting, throwing, catching, crouching, jumping, reaching, turning, twisting, squatting etc.

Everyday examples may be:
- Picking up a bag or child.
- Opening a door.
- Putting on clothing (socks, shoes, tops).

Your breath will protect your body by relaxing it as you move. Holding your breath brings tension and pressure into the body. The exhale, just like a sigh, relaxes it. This will:

- Protect your muscles from strain as you move throughout the day.
- Relax your body giving you more energy and economy of effort.
- Start to bring ease and pleasure to your movement.

TIP. *The best way to build a habit is to immediately correct yourself when you err. So if you stand up holding your breath, sit down and do it again correctly. You will then correct this bad habit in no time at all.*

To view the free video of this practise please use the link below: http://www.matthill.co.uk/living-systema

The Balance Set.

Balance is a crucial skill to a human being. Without good balance, performance in any sport or physical activity becomes a much harder prospect. Balance brings steadiness, calm, agility, poise and precision. It also brings physical confidence, which in turn brings psychological confidence.

Our balance is probably best for most of us when we are in childhood. This is mainly because we are always using our balance at this age. Children will always find things to balance across or on. Playing in the woods or the park provides lots of opportunities for balance. There is no reason why as adults we cant be doing the same thing. Also children don't have the fear of falling over that we do as we age. The ground is familiar territory to them.

As we age we become very brittle in our movements. We really begin to fear the ground, and with no wonder. The latest statistics from the Centre for Disease Control (CDC) in the US show that older age falls are the leading cause of injury and death in old age (people over 65). As people age they are aware of just how damaging a fall can be. The more they fear it, the more rigid and stiff they become. The more rigid and stiff they become, the more likely they are to not only fall, but to injure themselves when they do fall. They become like Mr. Glass in M. Knight Shaymalan's film, 'Unbreakable'.

Balance has strong links to confidence. As your balance improves, your confidence will also improve. Not just confidence in your physical ability but also your general confidence. In my experience there is a close correlation between confidence and a good general level of physical skill, a key part of which is balance.

Balance of course is much broader than just physical balance. Everything needs balance. You need balance within your body, diet, training, mind, day, family, life, it goes on. In fact, I would go as far as to say that balance is one of the most important concepts we have.

The good news is that balance can be improved at any age. Improve your leg strength through your entire range of movement and practising balance will improve your skills.

The next set of practises can be used as a good aid to improve balance.

To view the free video of this practise please use the link below: http://www.matthill.co.uk/living-systema

14. Ablutions on one leg.

This is an old Physiotherapists tool. It is simple and the great thing about it is that everybody (hopefully) will do this twice a day without fail.

When you do your ablutions, washing your face and brushing your teeth, do it standing on one leg. Do the bottom row standing on one leg and then the top row standing on the other. You want to be able to do it without hopping all over the bathroom.

Have the knee slightly bent; stand in good posture, relaxed and breathing. The good thing is that you are doing something else (brushing your teeth) **whilst** standing on one leg. This will get you used to developing the skill whilst multi tasking. I.e. while life goes on around you.

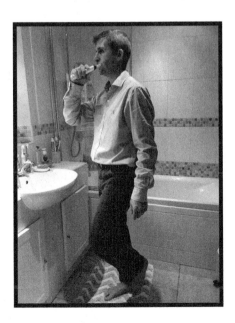

When you can do it comfortably try changing it up a little. You can for example change the angle of the standing leg. Try it with the foot:

- Facing in,
- Facing out,
  Standing on the ball of your foot,
- Standing on the outside (supinated),
- Standing on the inside (pronated) and,
- The (very difficult) heel.

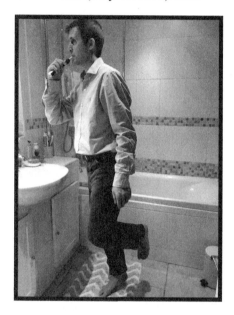

When you can do these variations, then try it with your eyes closed. This is advanced and comes with a warning. You are likely to wobble and fall, so please make sure that you are not going to injure yourself if you fall against something, or into the bath for instance. You could maybe try doing it in a corner or next to your bed for example.

To view the free video of this practise please use the link below: http://www.matthill.co.uk/living-systema

15. Use your feet.

This was a tip that Mikhail gave to Vladimir in order to improve his kicking ability. As you go about your daily routine in the house, try to do as much as you can with your feet. Try to:

- Open your underwear drawer and take out your socks and underwear with your foot.
- Open the bathroom door with your feet.
- Turn on the tap with your foot.
- Get your toothbrush with your foot.
- Get the towel off the rail with you foot.
- Open the other doors all the way down stairs with your feet.
- Open the drawers with your feet.
- You get the idea. Within reason, try as many things as you can during the day with your feet.

Key points:
- Try to use both feet, not just your good one.
- Be careful of falling.
- Be careful of damaging furniture (drawers, plates, rails etc.)

Benefits:
- You will improve balance.
- You will improve your foot and leg dexterity.
- You will become more supple (think about reaching door handles, toothbrushes etc.

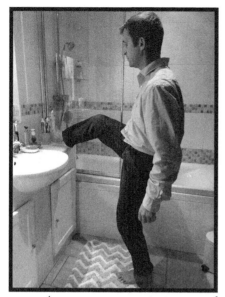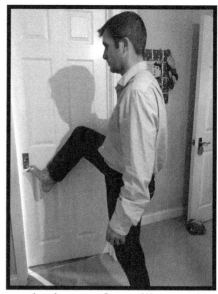

- As you use your toes more the muscles in your foot will strengthen, making you more stable and resilient to foot injury.

To be really dexterous, you need to do this barefoot of course. This gives you much more time spent barefoot. This massages the muscles of your feet and allows the bones of your feet to spread more in a very natural way. Our feet spend far too much time confined. Allowing them to breathe and spread is very healthy for them.

You can make this as challenging or as easy as you like. I bet however, that you will start pushing yourself.

To view the free video of this practise please use the link below: http://www.matthill.co.uk/living-systema

16. Put your shoes and socks on while standing up.

This is another action that we all do at least twice per day. When you make it a balance exercise, you find a great way to integrate training inside everyday actions.

It is simple.

In the morning, before and after training and whenever you enter and leave the house, you probably take at least your shoes off. When you do, you probably either sit or kneel down, or lean against something. Instead of this, just stand on one foot. Raise your other foot, unlace your shoe, remove it and smoothly place the foot down. Do the same with the sock if necessary and then do the same on the other side.

Again this is better than the exercise of just balancing on one foot because:
1. You are multi tasking, thereby making it more real.
2. It is not taking up extra time in your day.

I have one student in his 60's who says that this practise has done more for his balance than any other practise that I have suggested.

As always make sure that you check the key elements of your balance:
- Knee slightly bent.
- Exhale as you lift your leg in order to relax yourself.
- Keep your posture as straight as possible.
- Keep your muscles relaxed.
- Keep the action smooth and not snatched or jerky.

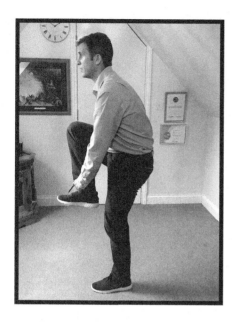

If you have to sit down to put your shoes and socks on or take them off then you are already old, whatever age you are!

To view the free video of this practise please use the link below: http://www.matthill.co.uk/living-systema

The Tension set.

Excess tension is a real problem for many people. Many are conscious of it and many are not. It can lead to all kinds of problems and ailments both mental and physical. I would go as far as to say that most people living a western lifestyle are too tense.

Surprised to hear this? No I didn't think so.

In order to think about tension, it is good to start with its opposite, relaxation.

The ability to relax is probably one of the most overlooked skills in life. All of the research shows that your ability to relax has a huge impact on your ability to deal with life and stress, to perform well, stay healthy and energized and to be creative.

Do you ever find everyday movements laborious and overly tiring? Many injuries and cases of fatigue come not from extreme exertion but from performing everyday movements with too much tension in our bodies.

Most movements that we do in the martial arts, sports or everyday life are easy. If you think of a punch, kicking, throwing or catching a ball, sitting down in a chair, lying down in bed to sleep, getting in and out of the car, picking up a bag, turning to look behind you when sitting down, walking, running or sitting at a computer, none of these are hard physical endeavours. However, for many people they can be laborious and cause discomfort, pain and fatigue.

The goal is to make these movements easy and graceful so that moving in sport, martial arts or everyday life becomes pleasurable, elegant and efficient, generating energy as opposed to being wasteful of energy.

Watch a world-class sports person or dancer. They make their movements look effortless and elegant. Think of Ali, George Best and Federer. Their ability to make the generation of speed, power and skill look effortless and smooth is legendary.

Sprinters for example, are widely known not for how well they can engage muscles but for how much of the race they can spend in relaxation. Think about how relaxed and effortless Usain Bolt makes sprinting look. As the great sprinting coach Charlie Francis puts it:

'The number one secret to greater speed is relaxation! It allows a faster and more complete shutdown of antagonists, quickening alternation cycles and permitting more force to be delivered in the desired direction with less energy consumption. **Relaxation must become second nature in every drill you do** *and every run you take. You may feel that you aren't generating enough force while relaxed (a perception that gets a lot of sprinters into trouble in big races), but remember; only the net force counts! The net force is the amount of force delivered in the desired direction, minus the force generated by the antagonist muscle at the same moment.'*

Much of the skill in making the impossible possible, the hard easy and the easy elegant, is down to how well you can relax individual muscles.

This is a skill. Most adults progressively lose their ability to differentiate parts of their body. I.e. to move or tense individual parts or muscles, whilst keeping others still or relaxed. For example, in many people the hips and lower back often move as one big block, causing forced unnatural movement and often resulting in strain and injury. There are some very simple movement exercises you can do to remedy this, to increase your freedom and range of movement.

Tension is contagious.

Skill in relaxation is also important to prevent an excess of tension in everyday life. When you sit at a desk typing you only need to be using your hands and fingers. However, the stress of work will often cause excess tension in surrounding muscles like your shoulders, neck, upper back and jaw. This causes headaches, fatigue and chronic injury. Keeping these muscles relaxed is a skill that can be developed.

Reducing tension in your movements will give you more energy, efficiency, power, smoothness, elegance, and timing. In effect it takes the brakes off. Moving with tension is like driving with the handbrake on.

Up to this point we have just dealt with physical tension. It is also important to relax your mental and emotional tensions. Relaxing your mental approach of always evaluating and thinking about situations and your responses to them, allows you to live and respond in a more spontaneous, natural and free way. Relaxing your emotional tension is vital for your health, energy and sanity. The breath is the key to this.

If moving with tension is like driving with the handbrake on, having too much emotional and mental tension is like *living* with the handbrake on.
Everyone from Steve Jobs to Einstein to Aristotle espoused the need to relax physically, mentally and emotionally in order to be creative. So whether you are looking for creativity in your job, business, hobby or spontaneous natural movement in your sport or martial art – work on how to be more relaxed, physically and in your approach.

My favourite actor, Antony Hopkins, puts it another way, "They talk [quoted] about relaxing, about being in charge of your instrument, being open to let the power flow through you.... You can't be tense. It's a whole principle of life. If you relax, good things will come to you. If you are uptight and aggressive, you frighten things away."

We carry around so many anxieties and worries. Stress comes into our lives in so many ways, and that stress causes tension in the muscles. An overload of tension will cause you:

- Loss of vital energy.
- Immobility and stiffness in the joints.
- Decreased circulation in the tense area.
- To lessen your ability to breathe smoothly, easily and deeply.

- Chronic muscle fatigue over time.
- Elevated blood pressure.

It will also lead to an elevated level of constant anxiety. The tension in the muscles actually locks in the emotion. It keeps the worries and anxieties there.

Luckily the opposite is also true.

When you learn to let go of your tension, you let go of the emotion that causes it.

You can achieve this by increasing your awareness on a moment-to-moment basis and having a few tools up your sleeve to learn how to release the tension.

The next few chapters will outline ways to do this.

To view the free video of this practise please use the link below: http://www.matthill.co.uk/living-systema

17. Tension Awareness.

At all times try to be aware of excess tension, whether sitting, standing or in motion, and drop it out with breathing and movement. One way to do this is to become aware of your breathing, or more importantly, your lack of breathing.

The other way is to listen to your body. If you are absent of tension, you will not feel your body (unless there is illness or injury). This level of moment-to-moment body awareness is a skill that can be developed. Many people are so used to constant pain that it becomes background noise. Don't settle for this. When you notice tension in your body, you need to move that part of your body.

We all carry around far more tension in our body than is needed. This practise is a great way to start noticing this during everyday activities, such as making a cup of tea (very British I know).

Use those moments when you are engaged in this kind of activity to exhale and relax your muscles. You will be amazed at how tense your shoulders, arms, neck, hips and legs etc. are. You want your muscles to be relaxed and hanging off the bones like water balloons, rather than holding your body up with tension like air balloons. You should strive to have only the amount of muscular effort in the body that it requires to do the work that it is doing.

This will help you to conserve energy, improve circulation and avoid chronic muscle strain and fatigue over time.

To view the free video of this practise please use the link below:
http://www.matthill.co.uk/living-systema

18. Tension and relaxation before sleep.

It is a great method to relax the body. Most people aren't aware of the tension levels in their body. In class when I ask people to relax their shoulders for example, they will say, "They are already relaxed!" I then say, "Ok tense your shoulders", and of course when they go to tense them they realise they are already tense.

This exercise is similar. When you are lying in bed, systematically go through your body tensing individual parts. This is a great exercise to do if you have trouble sleeping, especially if you are wound up tight from the day. It will systematically find your tension and release it. This is difficult to do in the early days, as it takes a while to get the body sensitivity to feel where you are carrying tension.

To begin the exercise lie on your back and begin with a few easy breath cycles. Inhales, exhales and maybe some light holds. Then, start with the left leg:

- Inhale and tense the left leg from the toes to the glutes.
- At this point, hold the breath and lightly wobble the rest of the body to check that it is not tense also. You will find that tension 'bleeds' into other areas. Isolating tension in your body is hard to begin with.
- Exhale and release all of the tension.
- Then do the right leg.
- Now do half the body - toes to waist.
- Then the left arm from fingers to shoulder.
- Then the right arm.
- Then do the torso, waist to neck.
- Then do the neck and head. Really screw the face up.

- Now do the other half of the body - waist to the top of the head.
- Now finally do the whole body. As you inhale, fill the body with tension from the toes to the head.
- Then as you exhale release the tension from the head to the toes.

Extra Bonus!

If you were able to do this, let's try to break the body into smaller parts. Try to isolate tension into the following areas using the same breathing method as above:

- Foot.
- Calf.
- Knee.
- Thigh.
- Hamstring.
- Glutes.
- Hand.
- Forearm.
- Bicep.
- Tricep.
- Shoulder.
- Stomach.
- Chest.
- Lower back.
- Upper back.
- Latimus (side) muscles.
- Front of the body.
- Back of the body.
- Left hand side of the body only.
- Right hand side of the body only.

These exercises will not only find and release tension; they will increase your proprioceptive (sense of the self in space) skills.

You will be able to identify and release tension from the body much faster and more effectively at any time thus:

- Increasing energy levels.
- Lowering blood pressure.
- Increasing metabolism.

- Boosting the immune system.
- Improving the lymphatic system.
- Improving the digestive system.

Also it goes without saying that although I have listed this as tension relaxation before sleep, it can of course be done anywhere, anytime. Just be careful when driving though, as there is a possibility that you may get a cramp while you are doing it.

To view the free video of this practise please use the link below: http://www.matthill.co.uk/living-systema

19. Continual small adjustments.

Become aware of when you are in a position for a long time. This could be when driving, stood in a queue, at your workstation, watching a game, out at dinner etc.

Without looking like you have ants in your pants, you want to make small movements. This will stop you seizing or stiffening up by spending too long in one position. You will be familiar with the feeling. When you have been in a car for hours and you arrive at your destination. You may get out to find that it takes you a few minutes before you can walk properly. Your body has literally taken the shape of the seat. It takes a while before your back, hips and hamstrings release enough for you to be able to walk straight. It should be clear to everyone that this is not good for you.

So while sitting you should make continual minor adjustments. Wiggle your hips, move your spine in a fish like shimmy, lift your shoulders and drop them, move your legs from side to side. Wobble the muscles in your thighs etc.

This will stop your body from stiffening up. To stop the fluids from pooling, you can also gently tense and release the muscles as per practise 18, but as mentioned just be aware of causing cramps that might affect your driving.

This is a great habit to get into. We are not designed to be still for more than about 20 minutes. You don't have to go crazy with this, but in this day and age, it is VERY easy to sit still for hours hardly moving at all.

To view the free video of this practise please use the link below:
http://www.matthill.co.uk/living-systema

20. Cultivate a playful attitude.

Whatever age you are, try to take the time to play, as often as you can. If you take your children or grandchildren to the park play on the apparatus with them. Play tag with your children and grandchildren (there is so much more than exercise here); go for a cycle ride or a swim with your them. Get down on the floor and play with your pet, roll around with your dog. If you are out on your own challenge yourself to run to the top of a hill, to hang from a tree branch, to run the length of a field, to roll down a hill. Anything you like. Just play. If you can, make sure it involves going to the ground and getting back up again.

It's the same with balance; find more ways to play with your balance skills. If

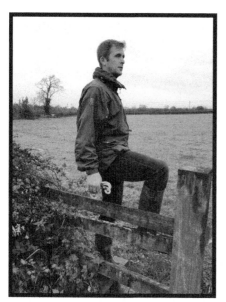 you have children play balancing games with them. Do challenges when you are out walking or playing in the park with them. Simple things such as who can stand on one leg the longest. If you have a dog, balance on things on your walk, it could be a kerb, log, wall or plank, whatever. Try to go over styles without using your hands.

However with all of these things, do not do it if you are not confident or feel that you may injure yourself. Just try to have the sense of playfulness that you

had as a child. Don't care about what people may think of you. You never know, you may just inspire someone!

Playing in the woods or even a children's play area will incorporate all or most of this. When was the last time you climbed a tree? Could you still do it? Here's a question: did most people stop doing these things because they couldn't do them anymore, or can they not do these things anymore because they stopped doing them? Getting older comes to us all, but in many ways getting older in terms of our ability to move well is a choice.

An attitude of play and fun in daily movement is vastly underrated. Remember 'exercise' is just a modern phenomenon of the past 40 years or so.

To view the free video of this practise please use the link below: http://www.matthill.co.uk/living-systema

Awareness Training.

The world of Systema, or indeed martial arts in general, is bigger than just the few moments of the fight. The fight starts way before it becomes physical. As an individual, we can safely say that if you are fighting, and didn't intend to be, you have missed the chance to do a lot of Systema in the build up. You were in the wrong place, with the wrong person or people, at the wrong time. In this day and age, if you find yourself in a fight, you have either been very unlucky, or you consciously or unconsciously missed a lot of chances to talk or walk your way out of it, or even better, avoid it in the first place. Your *situational awareness* of the location, person, atmosphere and yourself were probably lacking in some respect. There are of course unfortunate circumstances that we can do nothing about, but in my experience, these are rare. Very rare.

Awareness training has a number of uses. We will all be aware of its professional uses in the fields of counter intelligence, military, police, security and others. These professions are generally in the business of keeping themselves and others safe and therefore the awareness is primarily 'threat' focused. This is in keeping with our innate survival instincts. These are instincts that we all possess and are available for use on a daily basis. They provide us with a gut feel, an intuition, feelings that unfortunately many of us have ignored and overruled for so long, that they have become background noise. We don't even notice them.

This is a big difference between a civilian and a professional. A professional is 'switched on' to these instincts and feelings. This is partly because of their training and partly because it is their job to be aware. A large component of awareness training therefore is to teach us to start listening to these instincts again through consciously practicing the skills and listening or feeling for the instincts. It also requires a little skill training to know what to be looking for.

These professions need to be aware of what is developing, what fits in the environment and pattern of people's behavior and importantly what doesn't. Their lives and the lives of others depend upon it. This requires an ability to stay focused and present. To notice those things that others miss. Not just to look but to 'see', and they are assessing everything that they see. Whether they are walking through a forest, waiting at an airport or walking down a street.

They will be noticing and questioning things. What is here that shouldn't be? What isn't here that should be? Why has that person got a heavy coat on in summer? Are people moving naturally? Are people all looking at their phones or looking around? Are the birds singing or are they quiet? Why does that couple look out of place sat there?

This skill isn't just appropriate for the above-mentioned professions. The ability to notice a threat a few minutes or even seconds before others do, can save your own life and that of your loved ones. In this current climate of terrorist attacks in cities, knife and gun crime on the rise and petty theft and muggings, having a greater level of awareness is a good idea.

There are a number of things that you can do that I will outline in the coming chapter:

- Establish a baseline
- Improve sensory skill
- Improve awareness
- Make a plan
- Move unseen
- Play awareness-improving games with children or to challenge yourself.

Establishing a Baseline.

Establishing a baseline is about knowing what an environment should feel like and what the people in this environment should behave like. This was much easier in times gone by. Our environment back then would have been less complex. We would have been more in tune with it and we would not have changed it quite so often. Let me elaborate:

- The environment would have been much simpler as there would not have been so much development, technology or numbers of people. Think of your local town, district or vicinity. Now compare that to a more medieval or primal time. The variables would have been dramatically different.
- Technologically there would not have been vehicles, unnatural sounds and so many different types of clothing etc. to confuse or diffuse the senses.
- There would also not have been so many people. We can safely say

that we would have known pretty much everybody in our vicinity pretty well. So new people coming in or changes in the behavior of existing people would have been easy to read.

My teacher, Vladimir Vasiliev, talked about establishing a baseline at the 2016 Systema Summer Camp in Canada. He didn't use that term, but the essence was the same. We worked on a lot of different terrains: open field, close forest, water, by day and night. Vladimir encouraged us to notice when we changed to a different terrain; for example when we walked off a field and into the forest. We were to stop and take a minute or so to check ourselves. Take a breath. Smell the air. What can you smell? When you breathe in to smell, it is a different breath. It is softer, less harsh, more sensitive. You notice things. You will be amazed at what you can actually smell when you become more conscious of it. Was there any effect on our heart rate? Blood pressure? Tone or tension in the muscles? Nervous system? If so, we were to work to restore and remove the tension.

He then asked us to spread that sensitivity out to check the feeling in the group. Had it changed? Was there more anxiety, excitement, calm? There is wisdom in crowds, like herds, especially their instinct when it comes to threats.

Finally, Vladimir asked us to spread that sensitivity outside the group and into the wider area. Are there other people outside the group, around camp? Is their focus on us, or are they going about their business? What did we sense around us in nature from the wind, the trees?

This is an important skill for a professional.

However, it is also valuable in everyday life. If you walk into a business meeting do you take the time to check yourself before you go in? Are you calm and prepared? What is the feeling when you enter the room? Is it tense, friendly, guarded? Most of us naturally take a gut feel. It's built into us. But how many of us are conscious of it, let alone adjust our actions according to it.

I think this is more important than ever. When you walk into a pub, a busy train station, get on a train, enter a restaurant, attend an event or just walk through a supermarket or down a street, are you sensitive to the perceptions you are getting?

If it doesn't feel right, do you have the courage to get off the train or walk out of the restaurant or club? This may just be the highest level of martial arts. This is the ability to sense a problem and leave safely with your family and friends, before you even need to deploy or test your skills.

So in establishing a baseline we take the pulse of the locality. We ask ourselves the question, "Does this feel right?" Are the people acting normally? Is anyone looking stressed, fearful or anxious? Are people looking around a lot, especially behind them? If people are absorbed in their phones, or seem to be in their own worlds, chances are the threat level is low.

So, what if our answer, when we listen to it, tells us that something is not quite right?

Actions on!
In the military you would strive to have a prepared response for an anticipated situation. We called these, 'actions on' or the action that you carry out when faced with a certain situation. You tried to think about what response you would take before the situation occurred so that when it did occur, you could react faster. In certain circumstances, this can save you precious seconds, which can mean the difference between life and death. Examples would have been, 'action on' encountering enemy on the route in to the target, at the target, during the withdrawal etc. There may be times when you want to lie low and not engage the enemy in a way that may compromise the mission. Visualising and mentally rehearsing these things in advance is proven to allow a faster response under pressure.

It is equally good to have a couple of simple, 'actions on' in everyday life. So, returning to our question above: what if our gut instinct tells us that something is not quite right?

Firstly, leave the area, if it is safe to do so.

If, as above, you have walked into a bar and the atmosphere is not good, just

100

turn around and leave. If you are in a park or busy shopping area and you get the feeling that something isn't right. Just leave, calmly and smoothly, without any fuss.

If the situation is more immediate and urgent, for example a knife, car or gun attack, do the following:

- **Escape**. As fast and clean as you can. Drop anything that you are carrying, as it will get in the way and slow you down. Find somewhere safe.
- **Hide**. If you cannot escape the area, hide somewhere. Don't hide in groups. Lock doors if you can and barricade them. Stay out of the way of any windows, stay low and keep quiet.
- **Report**. Put your phone on silent and turn off vibrate. Rehearse how to do this now. Report the incident into the emergency services. Think of the six 'w's:
  1. Who you are?
  2. What happened?
  3. Where did it happen?
  4. When did it happen?
  5. Who is involved – who is the attacker – were they alone? What did they look like?
  6. Who else is involved? How many people are involved in the attack? How many people injured? How many people were in the room/area?

These are of course extreme cases, but try not to let the first time that you are faced with them be the time that you have considered them. Seconds count. In most cases the faster you can act the better your chance of survival. If you have mentally rehearsed a situation, you will react faster.

Building the skills – Childs Play

It is of course very difficult to maintain this level of awareness as an everyday Joe Blogs. When it is your job you have the training and the reason why. As an ordinary person, one of the hardest things about staying alert and aware is finding ways to stay 'switched on', concentrated and focused.

An effective way is to apply strategies or 'games' to it. There is nothing childish about this. It is the way that cultures have taught for generations. It is how sports emerged. Sports were of course originally ways for communities and then armies to prepare young men and then soldiers for battle during times of peace. Building games around natural survival and fighting skills is normal and natural. Importantly it is also great fun.

Whatever your age, these games, will make the practise of increasing your awareness and listening to your gut, more engaging, fun and will also add some useful skills to your arsenal. They are practical, fun and a way to get children out from in front of the TV.

They will also build in you and your children an increased sense of awareness, mindfulness and ability to not just look but **see** and act on what is going on around them.

Like so many tribal skills such as hunting, tracking, fighting, scouting, escaping etc. these skills were a natural part of life and learning when we lived in woods and forests. In basic children's games such as hide and seek and tag we had the makings of the warrior, who was aware, calm, fit and ready to act in a flash.

In the coming section I will introduce you to some games. Some, I am sure, will be old favourites, some will be new. Here is the list of activities:
1. 10 seconds to hide.
2. Exit Interview.
3. What do they do?
4. Professional eyewitness.
5. What's that sound – blindfolded?
6. What's that smell?
7. Observe and notice a list of things.
8. KIMS game.
9. Move without being noticed.
10. Stalking.

Game 1: 10 seconds to hide.

Aim:

The aim of this game is to hide from line of sight while still being able to see the target. To see without being seen. It is good to call this game randomly. Sometimes if we are out walking in a wood I will unexpectedly shout to my children, "10 seconds to hide!" and they have to react fast and get straight into the game.

Rules:

The watcher calls 'hide'. Everyone else has ten seconds (this can be varied depending on availability of cover) but it needs to be a short time frame. The watcher closes their eyes as they count. The watcher then opens their eyes, and staying in the same place, has to find the runners. It is important that the runners can see the catcher from their hiding position.

Where to play:

It is good to build this skill in any environment. Woodland, sand dunes, street, shopping centre, a house, anywhere you may need to run quickly from a threat and find cover.

Variations:

You can do this as a 'stalk'. I.e. the catcher stands in a location for example in a field of long grass, at the top of a hill or sat in a café and the runners have to get as close as they can without being seen.

In the beginning you can also do it so that the runners just have to hide and it doesn't matter if they can or can't see the watcher.

Specific skills being developed:

- Ability to find a hiding place quickly
- Ability to react quickly at unexpected moments.
- Ability to look through cover and see the target without being seen yourself.
- Observation and scanning skills.
- To be naturally scanning and noticing good hiding/ambush spots.

Game 2: Situational Observation.

Aim:

The aim of this game is to be able to successfully answer observational questions after leaving a location.

Rules:

In the beginning, tell participants in advance that they are going to play the game, so that they take notice. However after a while, they should be naturally more aware and be able to play it without prompting.

Upon leaving the location, e.g. a restaurant or play area, maybe on the walk or car journey home, you then ask a series of questions such as: How many pushchairs were in the play area? How many swings? What colour was the slide? Or in a restaurant, what drink did Bob drink? How many people were serving behind the bar? What colour was the carpet? What flowers were on the table? How many exits were there? Where would have been the safest place to sit and why? If a bad person/threat came in and you had to hide, where would you go?

Where to play:

Literally anywhere, restaurants, visits to a friend's house, days out at a museum, library, cinema, a walk etc.

Variations:

Over time you can start to ask more tactical questions such as, where would have been the safest place to sit? Where was the closest exit to us? Who was wearing clothes that could best have concealed a weapon of some kind? Who was acting strangely? Who looked out of place?

Specific skills being developed:

- Observation.
- Seeing rather than just looking.
- Memory and recall.
- Observation skills in the questioners.
- Observation and scanning skills.
- Looking for things that seem out of place or don't make sense, i.e. things/people that were there but shouldn't have been, or weren't there but should have been.

Game 3: What do they do?

Aim:
The aim of this game is to use observational skill to guess what a person does for a living. This will cultivate a more curious and critical mind in the participants.

Rules:
'People watch' someone for a few minutes. Then deduce what they do for a living. Notice things like their clothing. Is it obvious? Is it a uniform? Is it a genre of uniform that may not have a logo on it like a suit? Are they local or visiting? What is their walk like? Do they have a confident, military bearing? Do they look physically strong from manual work? Is their hair long or short? What about their hands? Soft? Hard from physical work? Is their physique a gym one or a manual work one?

It doesn't matter too much in the beginning whether you are correct, but that you are noticing and making sensible deductions. After a while you can begin to find out if you are correct.

Where to play:
Almost anywhere there are people that you can observe for a short period of time. Restaurants, coffee shops, airports, sat on a bench with people walking past etc.

Variations:
You can also work it the other way and try to look for a manual worker, office worker, local person, visitor etc. in a crowd.

Specific skills being developed:

- Observation.
- Ability to make sensible deductions based on observations.
- Seeing rather than just looking.
- Starting to notice and ask yourself questions about people, leading to noticing when people are out of place in an area and potential threats.

Game 4: Professional Eyewitness.

Aim:

The aim of this game is to give a detailed physical description of a subject. Again this will cultivate critical observational skills.

Rules:

Pick a person out. It could be someone who comes to your door or a waiter or waitress who comes to your table in a restaurant. It is best if you can take in the whole person.

Then pick someone to describe the visitor in detail. Try to use these categories:

- Physical: weight, height, age, hair and skin colour, ethnicity, left or right-handed, hairstyle, eye colour, and identifying features such as scars, freckles, tattoos, etc. build, gait, do they have a stoop, limp, are they fidgety?
- How about their voice, is it: smooth, rough, educated or uneducated? Is their speech accented? Do they use slang? Do they have a speech impediment? Try to get as much detail as you can.

A good way to remember this is A-H. **A**ge, **B**uild, **C**olour, **D**istinguishing features (carrying anything e.g. handbags rucksacks etc.), **E**levation (height) (handbags etc.), **F**ace, **G**ait, **H**air.

Where to play:

Again, almost anywhere there are people that you can observe for a short period of time. Restaurants, coffee shops, airports sat on a bench with people walking past etc. You could also do it on a TV programme.

Variations:

You can also work it the other way and describe in detail a specific person who you know is in the area that they have to look for. Alternatively you can give a 'type' of person for them to find.

Specific skills being developed:

- Detailed observation
- Starting to look deeper and deeper into a subject.
- Starting to notice and ask yourself questions about people leading to noticing when people are out of place in an area and potential threats.

Game 5: What's that smell?

Aim:

The aim of this game is to correctly guess a number of smells accurately in order to enhance your primary sense. The sense that is your first line of awareness and defence. Your sense of smell.

Rules:

A person is blindfolded (this can also be done with a line or group of people). You then pass a number of objects under their nose and they have to guess what the object is by the smell.

Examples of smells are:

Smoke, a burnt match, garlic, coffee, cut grass, leaves, ashes, polish, oil, petrol, onion, olive oil, tea, whisky, leather, boot polish.

Where to play:

Literally anywhere.

Specific skills being developed:

- Olfactory sensitivity.
- Recall.
- Brain stimulation.
- Stimulation of the primary alerting sense.

Anecdote:

The sense of smell is interesting. It was once primary, just like animals. If we go into the right environment, it returns to being our primary sense too.

In 2001 I was doing Jungle Training in Belize, Central America. I had been in the Jungle for about 6 weeks with B company 2PARA. I was sitting on my hammock, cleaning my weapon, when I caught a smell. I followed my nose up and my head moved left and right as my nose triangulated the smell. I could smell 'clean.'

You have to understand that after a number of weeks, myself and the other paratroopers were purposefully starting to smell like the Jungle. We didn't wash with soap, we just rinsed in the river. We had blended with our environment. So anything new coming in stood out immediately.

I later found out that there had been a change around in some of the local training team and a new guy had arrived. I could smell him from about 800m away. I was both amazed and heartened to know that we are only ever a few weeks away from returning to our innate abilities. In the Jungle our sense of sight wasn't as good at alerting us, with such density of vegetation you can rarely see that far in the Jungle. So our sense of smell very quickly became the primary sense once more.

Game 6: What's that noise?

Aim:

This one is similar to the previous game. The aim of this game is to correctly guess a number of noises accurately in order to enhance your auditory senses.

Rules:

The person is blindfolded. You then generate a number of noises using everyday objects or using your phone.

Examples of noises are:

Thunder, different animals, striking a match, rustling in a pocket, unzipping a bag, opening the popper on a pocket, opening a bag, cracking an egg, footsteps,

If you are thinking more tactical you can use:

Loading a magazine, making ready, taking a safety catch off, taking a knife out of its sheath, drawing a bow etc.

Where to play:

Literally anywhere. The car is a good idea as long as the driver isn't the one generating the sounds! I am sure there are some good apps for this.

Variations:

You can do this in different environments too and use the smells of that environment for example woodlands, beaches, cities etc.

Specific skills being developed:

- Auditory sensitivity
- Recall
- Brain stimulation.
- Stimulation of one of the primary alerting senses.

Game 7: Observe and notice a list of things.

Aim:

On a journey or visit, you have to look out for a list of items. This is ideal to keep children occupied on a journey. The winner is the first person to find all of the items.

Rules:

The list is pre-made. The person has to notice the item and tick it off the list. It can be done in groups or as individuals. You can also play this as the first person to spot the item claims it. The others have to wait until they see the item again.

Examples of objects are:

Red car (or any colour), bridge, church, person in a hat, farm animal, tractor, airplane, traffic light etc.

It is good also to start to look deeper. You can go for emotions or types of people such as a foreign language speaker, an angry person, a pregnant person, a brother or sister together, a depressed person, someone who has just got some bad news, someone up to no good etc.

Where to play:

Literally anywhere. Journeys, visits, even a dinner party or BBQ can be made more interesting by having to probe deeper into people and things.

Variations:

You can play a variation as more of a memory game where you allow people to memorise the list and then mentally check things off.

You can also do this in different environments too and introduce them to different types of things in those environments such as flora, fauna, life etc. in nature, or towns and cities. If on holiday in a foreign language speaking country it is a good way to learn the language by using the foreign names for objects.

Specific skills being developed:
- Observation skills.
- Memory skills if there is not a written list.
- Discernment skills.
- Being able to 'see' rather than just look.

Game 8: KIMS Game.

Aim:

This is a game that I first played on my Jungle Warfare Instructors Course. The aim of this game is to get sight of a number of objects for a short time of say 60 seconds. The objects are then covered up and you have to remember as many as possible.

Rules:

The objects are placed on a surface and then covered up. They are then revealed for a certain amount of time. No notes are allowed to be taken. The objects are then covered over again and you have to remember as many as possible. Set a certain time frame e.g. 5-10 seconds per item for the recall. As they get better you can drop that to 1-3 seconds for each item. You then have to recite as many as possible in that time frame.

Memory Techniques.

In ancient times, memory techniques were used to remember lists of items. The Greeks and Romans orators were very good at these. The famous Roman Orator Cicero, referred to it in his work *'De Oratore'*. They are good systems to review. They use a set series of *'loci'* or places in your imagination that remain constant. It could be a familiar street, a room in your house, or an imaginary 'palace' that you have constructed in your imagination. You then 'walk' the room, street or palace in your head and link the items that you want to remember with the existing landmarks or 'loci' in your head.

The key is to make the links memorable. Changing the size, colour, or interactions of the two helps to make the link more memorable. Examples are the 'Roman Room', the 'peg system'; the 'journey system' and Matteo Ricci's 'memory palace' made famous in Thomas Harris 'Hannibal' series of books.

Where to play:
Anywhere.

Variations:
You can also play a version where one object is taken away and they observers have to correctly identify which object has been removed.

Another version is to substitute an object e.g. one brand of matchbox for another or simply a matchbox for a lighter.

Specific skills being developed:
- Observation skills.
- Memory skills.
- Eye for detail.
- Memory techniques.

Game 9: Move without being noticed.

Aim:

This is not a game so much as an everyday activity. See if you can approach a group of people or remove yourself from a group without anyone acknowledging or noticing you.

The key is to move smoothly, not in a jerky noticeable manner, not too slow and not too fast.

You should be able to do it in everyday situations and not stand out as doing anything strange.

The people can be known to you or unknown. You will soon know if they have noticed you, as they will look at you or acknowledge you.

Try different angles such as approaching or leaving from the side, back, acute angles etc.

Also think about the timing. Try to approach or leave when they are distracted either in conversation, looking at something, or maybe an action such as tying a shoelace or opening a wallet.

The reaction you want them to have is, "When did so and so leave?" Or, "Wow when did you get here?"

Also notice when the same thing happens to you. If you suddenly notice someone has left or arrived without you noticing, you should mark how it happened. What were you doing at the time? How do they move? Is there anything different about it? Where are they stood in relation to you?

Note: The real key to this is to able to, 'disappear inside yourself'. You have to be able to clean yourself of tension, intention and be completely normal. If you have an intention of sneaking up, people will feel it. You have to be able to empty your intentions internally as well as in your movements.

Where to play:
Anywhere.

Specific skills being developed:
- Movement skills.
- Observation skills.
- Taking opportunities.
- Awareness.

Game 10: Stalking.

Aim:

This is an archetypal activity used by all cultures. The aim is to get as close as possible to 'prey' prior to delivering the final shot.

Rules:

Firstly agree the, 'playing area'. Agree the boundaries. For example you can do it in a valley. The 'prey' sits at the top of the valley and the 'hunters' try to stalk the prey who is static. The hunters' job is to get close enough for a bowshot or stones throw away, without being seen by the prey.

Both the hunter and prey are building skills. The prey is building the skill to watch, listen, predict routes and observe ground.

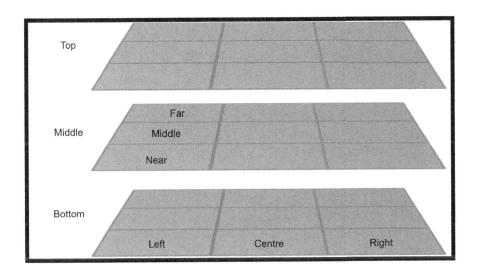

Observing Ground.

When observing ground it is good to use a grid system. Divide the ground into 9 rough squares, left, centre, right and near, middle far.

If there is canopy of trees or buildings it can be divided further into 9 squares when you include low, middle and high. That would then be 27 squares in total:

The hunters learn to move smoothly, silently and with patience, choosing good routes and being able to 'see' that route all the way to the target.

Where to play:

It is good to try this in different terrains. Woodland, urban, shops, desert, beach etc. Terrains that favour the hunter, such as thick woodland, or terrains that favour the prey, such as open fields or beach.

Variations:

You can also play this game with a moving 'prey'. So, much like a deer, the prey can move and the hunter(s) must move accordingly.

You can also play this in a supermarket or shopping mall as a fun variation.

Specific skills being developed:
- Movement skills.
- Observation skills.
- Stealth skills.
- Patience.

Annex 1: Are human beings compatible with 21st century living?

In short, no. From a physical standpoint and to thrive as human beings, we are designed to move much, much more. In our current lifestyle we spend most of our waking hours sitting. Think breakfast, then commutes, then office work, then commuting back, then dinner, then TV, and then bed. Nearly all of that is done in a seat.

We are not designed to sit that long and when we do, we get problems. We seize up, physically and psychologically (stress).

Rewind back to tribal living, where most of our time as human beings has been spent, and none of that would have been done in a seat.

We are designed for a day filled with walking, running, jumping, swimming, diving, hanging, swinging, rolling, squatting, twisting, pushing, pulling, lifting, throwing, getting down and up from the floor.

Playing in the woods or even a children's play area will have all or most of this. When was the last time you climbed a tree? Could you still do it? Here's a question: did most people stop doing these things because they couldn't do them anymore, or can they not do these things anymore because they stopped doing them? Getting older comes to us all, but in many ways, getting older in terms of our ability to move well is a choice.

Some of the best fun my three children had over Christmas was challenges I set them on dog walks for tree climbing.

Don't mistake this for high intensity exercise at the gym though. All this was done countless times during the day in the course of everyday life. An attitude of play and fun in daily movement is vastly underrated. 'Exercise' is just a modern phenomenon of the past 40 years or so.

In order to *thrive* as healthy normal human beings, we need to be moving our body through as big a range of movement as possible, every day. We should be able to do the four pillars through the full range of motion as a minimum. I would also add a fifth pillar, a pull up but brachial i.e. overarm not underarm chin up. The vertical hang is also fantastic for fixing shoulder problems (see *'Shoulder Pain, The Solution And Prevention' by Professor John Kirsch MD.*)

When we can move well, we are able to enjoy life much more fully. It also cleans us out psychologically. We literally move and breathe stress and anxiety out of our bodies. It gets locked and hidden in our bodies when we spend too much time thinking and worrying while sitting still, in stasis, and we need to move through our whole body to find stiffness, tension (stress) and ease it out.

For the best results try not to limit yourself to just one type of activity such as running, cycling or swimming. Humans are all-rounders. There are better runners, jumpers, climbers, swimmers etc. in the animal kingdom, but we are the best all-rounders. So try to find something with lots of varied movement. If you are too specific in your type of movement, you will pay a price (balance in your body, injury and boredom).

As this book has hopefully shown you it is quite easy to incorporate these movements into everyday life and feel the benefits very quickly.

Annex 2: My Daily non-negotiables.

These are things that I think that you have to do everyday. They are not overly onerous, but when you attain a basic standard, you will have a body that will be strong enough and mobile enough to get you through life smoothly and easily. My key daily non-negotiables are:

1. Do one of each pillar.
2. Get down to the floor and back up again.
3. Walk.
4. Get outside, preferably in a natural environment.

One of each pillar.

The five pillars together check the whole body. They check that:

- You are strong enough to move your body slowly and smoothly through its full range of motion.
- You are able to breathe continuously throughout the motion without your breath getting strained or stopping completely.
- You are flexible enough to move through your natural range of motion, especially the leg raise and the squat.

The rub is that you have to do each pillar slow, ideally as slow as you can. This means taking about 30 seconds down and 30 seconds up if you can for each of them. Admittedly this may be tough for the pull up. In this case you can do each of the phases slightly separately. Pull up as slow as you can (you probably wont get your chin over the bar this way) and then come down and jump into the pull up so that you get your chin over the bar and lower down slowly.

Get down to the floor and back up again.

I talk about this a lot. One of the big differences between the old and the young is their ability to get smoothly to the floor and back up again without effort or strain. Don't become a stranger to the floor as you age. The idea is that if you do it every day, there will not come a time when you can't do it. This is especially important as we age. Falls kill more people in old age than cancer, heart attacks or any other health issue. Many who fall never make it back out of hospital and many cannot even get themselves back up after falling. Learning to get smoothly to the floor and back up again, without pressuring the system is hugely important. In fact I would go as far as to say that it is a critical life skill.

Daily constitutional

It's about so much more than A-B or even calorie burn.

When I first talk about relearning your walk at Systema classes, I can see people looking at me dubiously. After all, they have been walking ok for their whole lives. The difference is that I want them to walk in a way that promotes health, not just in terms of calorie burn, but also in terms of resetting the system and removing stress.

Walking is the defining movement of a human being and the great thing about walking, is that you can't be sitting at the same time.

Few people in the western world walk enough these days and the benefits are well documented:
- Calorie burn.
- Endorphin release (mood enhancers).
- Tones the muscles.
- Strengthens the heart.
- Reduces risk of diseases such as diabetes and cancer.
- However, you can get more.

Walking is our natural reset button. We know this intuitively. When someone is stressed or angry we say to them, "Come on lets go for a walk."

Adding just a few elements to improve your walking can enhance the effects stated above. Daily life puts stress in our bodies. Physical stress from sitting too much, bad posture, high stress lifestyles etc. This is compounded by emotional stress which starts as a thought or worry and quickly becomes physical tension in the body.

Walking is our natural antidote to this. When walking correctly you literally breathe and walk the stress out of your body.

Here are a few steps to help this.

Focus on your breathing. Try to link it to your steps. Breathe in through your nose for say 4 steps and then out through your mouth for 4 steps. As you relax and improve, you can stretch this to 6, 8, 10 or more. You then also get all the benefits of nasal breathing that I have outlined before.

Relax on the exhale. As you exhale, try to relax your muscles from the head down to the feet. Your body should feel light. In fact, your body should 'disappear'. If you are relaxed and in good posture, you should not feel your body. All you should feel is the contact of your feet on the floor.

Walk from the knees. This will relax your leg muscles, make you more energy efficient, lighten your step reducing impact and make you more balanced over uneven terrain. To do this, begin the step by relaxing and moving the knee forwards.

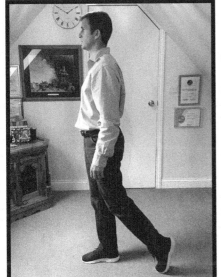

Maintain a good posture. Chin should be in and pulled back, chest should be out and not sunken, arms loose and relaxed at your sides. Key is not to pull your shoulders back, but to lift your chest gently out in a way that does not add tension to your muscles. This will ensure that you are not building tension and pain through bad posture.

It obviously helps to walk outside in fresh air, preferably in proximity to trees. When you walk with these four points in mind, you will amplify the benefit of getting outside and dosing up on vitamin D.

Just like a computer that has to process too much and needs to be reset, our natural reset is walking. In a very short space of time we can switch off and then on again using walking and keeping these points in mind.

Get outside

Obviously this can be done in conjunction with the previous non-negotiable of walking. I think that it is so easy to underestimate the need to get outside. Whatever the weather (important in the UK!) you should get out and spend time getting daylight on your skin. At minimum 20 minutes. Walk, work in the garden, drink tea, have lunch or dinner. Or, shock, horror, just sit and do nothing for twenty minutes. Breathe fresh air and just sit with your own thoughts. No phone, or even a book. You will be amazed what comes to you. In fact, just sitting was going to be another of my non-negotiable, but I thought that just sitting, as opposed to doing pillars, would be a step to far for many of you!

Annex 3 - The Benefits of Nasal Breathing and Breath Ladders.

Excerpt taken from Systema Health, 25 practises for a lifetime of health and wellbeing.

In life, the very first thing that we do is inhale and the last thing that we do is exhale. Every moment in between, involves breathing. A better understanding of your breathing, and practice in mastering it, can create dramatic changes in the quality of your life.

There are three phases of breath. Inhale, exhale and hold. We will deal with all three in this section.

In Systema there are three basic things to remember when it comes to breathing.

1. Inhale through the nose.
2. Exhale through the mouth (when under physical or mental stress or strain) and;
3. Don't stop or hold your breath.

You will be amazed when you notice just how often you hold your breath. You will probably hold your breath when doing something even mildly strenuous, like sitting down or standing up. When thinking or concentrating, or when taken by an emotion such as fear or surprise. The key aim of correct breathing is to calm and relax you. There are also some real health benefits to breathing correctly through the nose, as opposed to the mouth:

- It filters the air catching dirt and dust particles on the nasal hairs and mucus membrane.
- It activates your immune system.
- It cools and optimises the pituitary gland, one of the main hormone production centers in the body.
- It warms the air to 35 degrees centigrade, the optimum temperature for the air to be absorbed through the lung wall and into the blood stream.
- It stimulates the body's production of Nitric Oxide (NO) gas, which is a natural relaxant and a cousin of laughing gas.
- It helps to keep the sinus passage clear to keep the brain cool and avoid sinus problems.
- It aids early detection of harmful substances
- It aids intuition and decision-making, we can smell fear and danger.
- It interrupts the panic cycle. When our thoughts start to escalate and spin out of control in times of high stress or danger, an inhale through the nose interrupts this and allows you to bring your breathing and thoughts back under control.

Finally and crucially, it activates the para-sympathetic nervous system, your rest and digest state. This is opposed to the sympathetic nervous system, your fight or flight state. By activating the para-sympathetic nervous system, we do several crucial things. We:
- Lower the heart rate.
- Lower the blood pressure.
- Relax the muscles.
- Allow for calmer, clearer thinking.
- Open up our senses (sight, sound) avoiding tunnel vision and the 'rushing or pounding' sound of blood in the ears.
- Normalise our perception of time, space and reason.
- We will cover three breath cycles to help you induce calm into your system: Circular breath, triangular breath and square breath.

BREATH LADDERS

Our natural 'reset' button

Breath ladders are a great way to practise walking and running, with minimal tension and with deep calming breaths. You learn to 'clean' yourself of tension as you move, so that your walk is stable and solid; neither floppy nor tense.

As with the prone breath cycles, you can do any breath pattern. A good start point is to try to go from 1 up to 10 and then back down to 1. So you inhale for one step, then exhale for 1 step. Then you inhale for 2 steps, exhale for 2 steps. Inhale for 3, exhale for 3. All the way up to 10 steps inhale and 10 steps exhale. Then you come back down 9, 8, 7 etc. all the way to 1. When you have completed this forwards, then try it backwards. You can also try it with the breath cycles shown in practise 1.

Combining your breathing and your walking is a critical stage to master early in Systema. It shows you how to recover yourself from stress and trauma and it also shows you how to keep movement in your body to aid recovery.

When the stress level is high, you should focus on one step inhale, one step exhale, gradually lengthening and smoothing out, as you calm the body, mind and emotions.

As you walk, subtly check your body for tension with movement of the shoulders, arms, hips, legs etc. Check that your muscles are not tight by wobbling them. If you can feel them wobble, it is a good indication that they are relaxed.

During the running stage, try to run in a way that relaxes all of your muscles. Vladimir Vasiliev states that there are traditionally only two reasons to run. Out of fear, and to relax. This is a run to show you how to relax. The arms are loose (imagine them as ropes tied to your shoulders with a heavy knot in the end. They should jangle as you run). Then try to get this feeling of looseness in the muscles into your whole body. You should be able to bring your attention to all muscles and joints in the body and feel them wobbling around as you run. Do the same breathing patterns with the running, as you did with the walking including going backwards.

IMPORTANT: It is important that you practice going backwards. When you first try this, you will be apprehensive about walking into something or falling over. Practise relaxing (especially the shoulders and hips) and try not to look over your shoulder. Go slowly, in a safe place and learn to relax. In a combat situation, you will probably spend as much time going backwards as forwards. Endeavor to get comfortable moving in a smooth relaxed manner in every way that you can.

Walking is a great 'reset button' for the body. Much like turning a computer off and then back on again when it freezes. Linking your walking with your breathing and focusing on relaxation, can be used to calm and restore your body, mind and spirit in times of need.

Conclusion.

A good friend recently said to me, "The best time to train, is when you haven't got time to train." I think that phrase sums this book up well.

Systema is a huge topic. If you only look at the fighting aspects of the art, you are at best studying only 20% of it. Your chances to practice it are also limited. However, if you open it up and think about practicing it in every moment, you can start to immerse yourself into it fully.

Also it is important to ask yourself, "What are the chances of me using Systema principles in a fight tonight, tomorrow, next week, this year, for the rest of my life?" The answer for most of us is probably, "Unlikely." However, if you ask how often you will use Systema principles as a parent, partner, friend or colleague or just in everyday movements, then the answer is, "definitely." This book is for those moments.

It is my hope that you will continue your exploration into Systema through the concepts outlined in this book over the coming months and years. To fully understand Systema, it has to become yours, not a copy of someone else. You have to allow the seed of Systema to germinate inside you and then grow out through your every breath, movement, thought, until it is naturally yours.

If you wish to progress further in your journey you should seek out a good instructor. Vladimir Vasiliev has a useful instructor search tool on his website: https://www.russianmartialart.com/schoollocator.php

Try not to get frustrated in your progress. I wish you fortune and strength in your journey. If you have any questions please feel free to contact me through the website www.matthill.co.uk or email matt@matthill.co.uk

Don't forget to get access to your complimentary video of each of the 20 practises outlined in the book by using this link:

http://www.matthill.co.uk/living-systema

Resources.

As Systema grows more and more resources are becoming available. It should be stressed again that nothing can replace a good instructor. What is the best way to find a good instructor? Look at their students. Vladimir Vasiliev's website has a great tool for finding instructors and clubs.

Recommended Reading:
Let Every Breath - Vladimir Vasiliev.
Strikes, Soul Meets Body - Vladimir Vasiliev.
Systema Health – Matt Hill
Systema Combat – Matt Hill

Recommended Viewing:
I have an online store of downloadable videos that can be found at: https://matthill.pivotshare.com/
Both Mikhail Ryabko and Vladimir Vasiliev have extensive video collections. Videos for both teachers can be found and purchased from their websites.

For free access to the 20 videos available for the practices outlined in the book use this link: http://www.matthill.co.uk/living-systema

CPSIA information can be obtained
at www.ICGtesting.com
Printed in the USA
BVOW05s0637151217
502854BV00015B/130/P